BICYCLING

For

LADIES

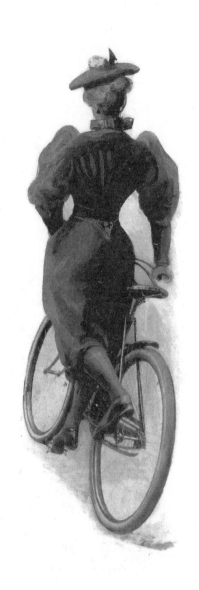

BICYCLING

FOR

LADIES

The Classic 1896 Guide to Skills,
Exercise, Mechanics, and Dress

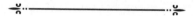

MARIA E. WARD

with Photographic Support by **ALICE AUSTEN**

APOLLO
PUBLISHERS

Bicycling for Ladies: The Classic 1896 Guide to
Skills, Exercise, Mechanics, and Dress

Bicycling for Ladies was originally published in 1896 and titled The Common Sense
of Bicycling, Bicycling for Ladies: With Hints as to the Art of Wheeling–Advice to
Beginners–Dress–Care of the Bicycle–Mechanics–Training–Exercise, etc. etc.
New design and text copyright © 2021 by Apollo Publishers

Apollo Publishers books may be purchased for educational, business, or
sales promotional use. Special editions may be made available upon request.
For details, contact Apollo Publishers at info@apollopublishers.com.

Visit our website at www.apollopublishers.com.

Library of Congress Control Number: 2020935830.

Published in compliance with California's Proposition 65.

Print ISBN: 978-1-948062-52-7
Ebook ISBN: 978-1-948062-53-4

Printed in the United States of America.

Contents

LIST OF
ILLUSTRATIONS

PREFACE

Originally published in 1896, Maria ("Violet") Ward's spectacular volume *Bicycling for Ladies* shocked and delighted a Victorian culture and gave women the tools they needed to master the art of bicycling, and thus have a road to autonomy. Today it remains comprehensive in explaining the basic components of the bicycle and how to ride one, and is also a delightful look back. This new edition, published more than a century after the first, maintains the original text and illustrations produced from photographs by the acclaimed photographer Alice Austen, as well as insightful and contextualizing forewords by Victoria Munro, executive director of the Alice Austen House, and

Maxine Friedman, chief curator of Historic Richmond Town in Staten Island, New York. Both the Alice Austen House and Historic Richmond Town own photographs and memorabilia related to Violet Ward and her family, Alice Austen, and Daisy Elliott, who modeled for the images in *Bicycling for Ladies*.

Maria E. Ward, known as Violet, and her circle of women friends who contributed to *Bicycling for Ladies* were in a league all of their own. They were trailblazers, breaking away from the constraints of their Victorian environment to forge independent lives that broke boundaries of acceptable female behavior and social rules.

The cover of the first edition of *Bicycling for Ladies*, published in 1896, is a rich blue with golden highlights depicting a woman at its center, wearing bloomers, kicking her feet forward with her hat flying off as she revels in cycling alone down a country road. This representation of independence and athleticism suggested the possibilities of new freedoms and exciting adventures for women in the Victorian era.

Ward celebrated this newfound independence in her writings, which moved beyond instruction of proper riding form to explore the mechanics of the bicycle and understanding the tools used to maintain and fix them. Sharing Ward's enthusiasm for new technologies was her close friend Alice Austen. Austen was a skillful photographer, and on a makeshift set on the lawn of her Staten Island home, she took the photos used to richly illustrate Ward's book. The model, Daisy Elliott, who shared Ward's and Austen's enthusiasm for sports, was a gymnast and a manager of a sports facility for women in Manhattan. She was also Austen's lover.

There have been various interpretations of *Bicycling for Ladies*, but few explore the importance of its illustrations and the social relationships of the women who collaborated to create this landmark book. Ward and her friends strived to be independent women who rejected traditional Victorian women's roles of marriage and motherhood. With her camera, Austen documented the connection between women's physical mobility and their personal freedom. Daisy Elliott is depicted here in strong athletic poses, as she is in several of Austen's other photography collections.

Austen was introduced to photography at age ten in 1876. A second-floor closet of her home on the shoreline of the New York Narrows Harbor served as her darkroom. In this home studio, which was also one of her photographic muses, she produced more than seven thousand photographs of a rapidly changing New York City, making significant contributions to photographic history by documenting Victorian women's social activities, New York's immigrant populations, and the natural and architectural world of her and her friends' travels.

One of America's first female photographers to work outside of the studio, Austen often transported up to fifty pounds of photographic equipment on her bicycle to capture her world. In Austen's letter archives there are several correspondences between Elliott and Ward and Austen from around the time of the *Bicycling for Ladies* publication, which reveal their adventurous travels and the intimate nature of their relationships. In an 1891 letter to Austen sent during her travels, Ward writes:

I only wish you were along, what fun we would have together. My camera is here and I hope to take back some work with me. Undeveloped of course. Did you succeed in securing some snow plates this year? What opportunities you must have had with this season of cold.

Elliott would write to Austen in 1897:

You know that I love you darling; there are many things I think of that I would like to do for you, yet, there is so little I really can. Whenever there is anything I could do, and don't, please let me know; because there is nothing [that] gives me more true pleasure than doing for one I love as I do you.

These women led incredibly full, liberated, nontraditional lives that could be the subject of several volumes of books. Understanding this makes the reading of this book all the more interesting and pleasurable. *Bicycling for Ladies* can truly be viewed as an early marker of the women's liberation movement and an important piece of lesbian history.

BICYCLING FOR LADIES: STATEN ISLAND AND THE BICYCLING CRAZE OF THE 1890s

A bright, sunny morning, fresh and cool; good roads and a dry atmosphere; a beautiful country before you, all your own to see and enjoy; a properly adjusted wheel awaiting you,—what more delightful than to mount and speed away, the whirr of the wheels, the soft grit of the tire, an occasional chain-clank the only sounds added to the chorus of the morning, as, the pace attained, the road stretches away before you!

So wrote Maria E. Ward in the first chapter of her book *Bicycling for Ladies*, published in 1896. The Staten Island native, known to her friends and family as Violet, was a vocal proponent of bicycling as an ideal outdoor sport for women, and her book came on the market precisely at the peak of bicycling's greatest popularity in the United States.

Teaching women how to ride a bicycle might seem an unusual topic to today's readers, but bicycling as a widely popular and affordable activity was barely ten years old in 1896. Early versions of the bicycle included the heavy "boneshaker" of the 1860s and the high wheelers of the 1870s and 1880s, but none of the early versions found mass acceptance, and most of those who did use them were men.

Bicycling changed dramatically in 1887 with the introduction of the "safety" bicycle to the United States. Featuring two wheels of equal size, and a chain drive that made riding more efficient, the new bicycle found quick acceptance among both men and women. The addition of pneumatic tires in 1889 gave a smoother ride, and assembly-line production lowered the cost. By the early 1890s, a bicycling craze was sweeping the nation, with millions of Americans enjoying the sport of "wheeling," as it was sometimes called.

While cycling was enjoyed by both men and women, it was women in particular who benefitted from this new activity. For the first time, it was considered socially acceptable for women to travel alone. Susan B. Anthony, a leader of the American women's movement, stated in an 1896 *New York World* interview that bicycling "has done more to emancipate women than anything else in the world. It gives women a feeling of freedom and self-reliance." Women reveled in this newfound freedom, joining bicycling clubs and participating in extended rides and country tours.

The popular acceptance of bicycling also had a dramatic and lasting impact on women's clothing. A dress-reform movement in the latter part of the 1800s sought to make women's clothing more practical and comfortable, and move away from the heavy and restrictive styles that impeded their ability to move freely. However, it was not until women took up bicycling that styles truly began to change. Riding a bicycle while wearing a tight-fitting corset and a long skirt was not only difficult but potentially dangerous, as the skirt's fabric could become entangled in the bicycle. Clothing manufacturers soon designed new bicycling outfits that offered such comforts as divided skirts, shorter skirt lengths, and lighter and less confining undergarments. The corset was on its way out, and clothing that allowed freedom of movement had come to stay.

BICYCLING FOR LADIES

Violet and her good friend Alice Austen, the noted photographer, took full advantage of the era's new sporting opportunities for women. They were avid tennis players as well as bicyclists, and numerous Austen photographs from the 1880s and 1890s captured scenes of both activities. Violet belonged to the St. Nicholas Skating Club in Manhattan, and was a member of the American Association for the Advancement of Physical Education. She also participated in the new enthusiasm for golf, with memberships in the Harbour Hills Golf Club of New Brighton and the Richmond County Country Club. In fact, correspondence and design drawings in the Historical Society's Ward family archival collection document Violet's efforts to patent a variation on a golf club.

But more than any other sport, it was bicycling that captured Violet's imagination. In 1895 she signed an agreement with the publishing firm Brentano's to publish *Bicycling for Ladies*. The agreement stated that Violet would receive 10 percent of the retail price for every copy sold in the United States, and 5 percent of the net price received for copies sold in Great Britain and other countries.

Violet's interest in the subject was all-encompassing. She described the bicycle as "an educational factor . . . creating the desire for progress, the preference for what is better, the striving for the best, broadening the intelligence and intensifying love of home and country." She praised the social benefits of bicycling, but was equally interested in human physiology and in the mechanical operation of the bicycle. Chapter headings included "What the Bicycle Does," "The Art of Wheeling on a Bicycle," "Position and Power," "Mechanics of Bicycling," and "Exercise." In the chapters "Women and Tools" and "Tools and How to Use Them," Violet made clear her belief that women were perfectly capable of maintaining and repairing their own bicycles: "I hold that any woman who is able to use a needle or scissors can use other tools equally well." She also addressed those who still believed that physical activities were not appropriate for women: "There is much prejudice against athletic exercise for women and girls, many believing that nothing of the kind can be done without over-doing," and continued on to explain that success was readily achievable with proper training and practice. Every chapter of the book gave evidence of Violet's unwavering conviction that women could, and should, lead physically active lives.

Violet clearly agreed with the new sensibility in women's clothing, and she devoted a full chapter of her book to describing what she considered to be the ideal bicycling outfit. "The combination of knickerbockers, shirt-waist, and stockings forms the essential part of a cycling costume," she wrote, along with shoes, gaiters, sweater, coat, hat, gloves, and an optional skirt. She went on to describe in detail the fabric, style, fit, and construction of each garment, with suggestions for accommodating the changing seasons. Most important, women's bicycling outfits "should have no constricting, no tight bands anywhere, but should permit of absolute freedom of movement. . . . Bicycling requires the same freedom of movement that swimming does, and the dress must not hamper or hinder."

To create the illustrations for her book, Violet teamed up with Alice Austen and their friend Daisy Elliott, a professional gymnast. Using draped fabric as a backdrop, Alice took a series of photographs as Daisy demonstrated the proper way for a woman to mount, pedal, and dismount a bicycle, as well as how to make repairs. The photos were then turned into hand-drawn illustrations for inclusion in the book, as the recent technological innovations that allowed for photographic reproductions in printing were not yet in widespread use.

The book received considerable notice upon publication. Reviews appeared in contemporary issues of *Book News*, *The Critic*, *The Book Buyer*, and *The Literary News*, among others. The reviewer in *Book News: A Monthly Survey of General Literature* commented that the book "is a serious and dignified discussion of the advantages of wheeling with hints as to its value, its proper enjoyment, the difficulties of beginning, the dress of the rider and the care of the wheel, with remarks upon exercise, training, etc." A reviewer in *The Publishers' Weekly: American Book-Trade Journal* took a lighter view, noting that "*Bicycling for Ladies*, by Maria E. Ward, profusely illustrated, is an altogether reliable and very pretty book, specially suitable for a young man to offer a girl who 'goes a-wheeling' with him."

Apparently pleased with the positive reception for her *Bicycling for Ladies*, Violet began to explore the possibility of another publication on the topic. In June 1896 she sent letters to a number of bicycle and tire manufacturers, explaining that she intended to "publish a work on component parts of bicycles, and chiefly on bicycle tires." She requested descriptions of each company's particular tire, and also solicited paid advertising from these manufacturers to offset the expense of the new publication. The advertising manager of the Pope Manufacturing Company, a major bicycle manufacturing firm, responded that they had received a copy of her book, and having "noted with much interest your clever work within," they would be "glad to have particulars of the larger work on this subject that you have in preparation." Other manufacturers, unfortunately, declined her invitation, and the second book was not published.

BICYCLING ON STATEN ISLAND

Violet Ward and Alice Austen shared their enthusiasm for bicycling with fellow Staten Islanders. Their names appear as the only two members of the Staten Island Bicycle Club's Executive Committee on a flyer dated June 1, 1895. The flyer notified potential members that after one successful season, the club had secured quarters in a building at the corner of Jay Street (now part of Richmond Terrace) and Wall Street in St. George. The clubhouse featured assembly rooms, locker rooms, a "wheelery" for bicycle rentals and repairs, and a storage room where "competent men will be in charge," should anyone wish to keep their bicycle in the building.

Along with serving on the club's Executive Committee, Violet Ward also took on the task of managing the new wheelery, named the Staten Island Bicycle Shop. In June 1895 she sent a letter to the Unadilla Tire Company, explaining that she was opening a bicycle store at St. George and would like to receive their catalog and wholesale price list. The Staten Island Historical Society's archives contains several invoices that show the equipment she purchased in September and October 1895 for the shop, including plugs, bolts, cement, springs, varnish, and pedals. An invoice from December 1895 records payment from a Mrs. Harding for repairing a puncture at a cost of one dollar.

At the time the Staten Island Bicycle Shop came into being, only five other bicycle businesses were listed in the Staten Island business directory. In 1898, the list of businesses under the heading of "Bicycles &c." was up to fifteen. It is not known how long the Staten Island Bicycle Shop remained open, but it does not appear to have been a long-lived operation.

By the early 1900s, on Staten Island and across the country, the vast enthusiasm for bicycling had waned. There are differing theories about why the bicycle craze passed, but many people credit the arrival of the automobile with bringing an end to the bicycle's heyday. In 1911, only six bicycle shops were listed in the Staten Island business directory, as compared with eighteen automobile dealers and repair shops. But Violet Ward and Alice Austen would no doubt be pleased to know that today bicycling is once again riding a wave of popularity, and that they were among the pioneers who helped pave the way.

THE COMMON SENSE OF BICYCLING

BICYCLING FOR LADIES

WITH HINTS AS TO THE ART OF WHEELING—
ADVICE TO BEGINNERS—DRESS—CARE OF
THE BICYCLE - MECHANICS—TRAIN-
ING—EXERCISE, ETC., ETC.

BY

MARIA E. WARD

ILLUSTRATED

New York:
BRENTANO'S

CHICAGO　　　　WASHINGTON　　　　PARIS

ORIGINAL TITLE PAGE SHOWING A DELIGHTFUL SUBTITLE, ETC., ETC.

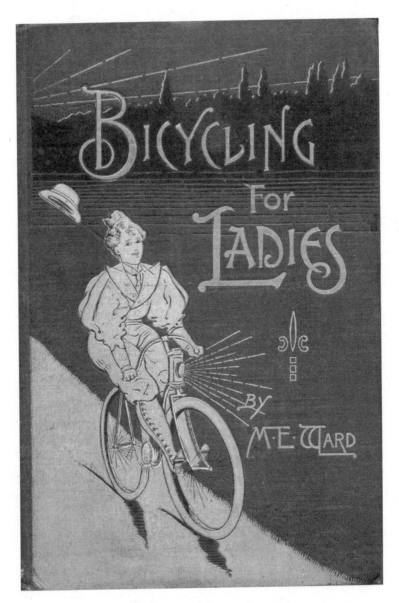

FRONT COVER OF ORIGINAL EDITION

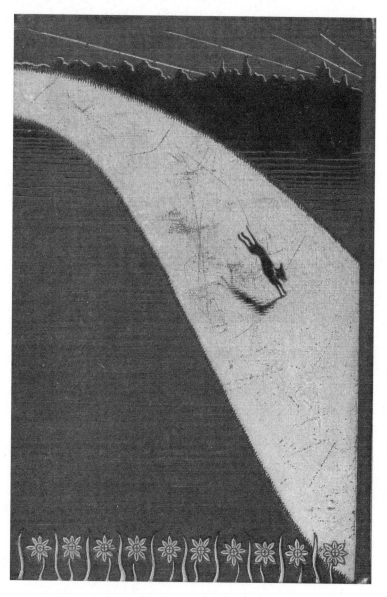

BACK COVER OF ORIGINAL EDITION

I have found that in bicycling, as in other sports essayed by them, women and girls bring upon themselves censure from many sources. I have also found that this censure, though almost invariably deserved, is called forth not so much by what they do as the way they do it.

It is quite natural to suppose, in attempting an unaccustomed exercise, that you have to do only what you see done and as others about you are doing. But to attain success in bicycling, as in other things, it is necessary to study the means as well as to look to the end to be attained, and to understand what must not be attempted as well as to know each step that will be an advance on the road to progress.

A great deal has been said against attempting to study a little of anything; but when a slight knowledge of several important branches of science that bear directly upon a subject under consideration, and that a subject concerning the health and safety of many individuals, will render one intelligently self-dependent, and able at least to exercise without endangering one's own health or the lives of others, the acquisition of such knowledge should not be neglected.

There are laws of mechanics and of physiology that directly concern the cyclist; it has been the author's aim to point out these laws, showing, for instance, the possible dangers of exercise, and how they may be avoided by the application to bicycle exercise of simple and well-known physiological laws, thus enabling the cyclist to resist fatigue and avoid over-exertion. The needs of the bicyclist are an intelligent comprehension of the bicycle as a machine, an appreciative knowledge of the human machine that propels it, and a realization of the fact that rider and bicycle should form one combined mechanism. For this, a knowledge of the laws that determine the limits and possibilities of both mechanisms is necessary. The cyclist is limited, not only by laws physiological and laws mechanical, which determine when and for how long he may travel, but he is restricted by the laws and ordinances of county, town and village as to how and where he may travel. A knowledge of these laws is also necessary.

While not attempting to treat any of these subjects exhaustively, the author has endeavored to place them comprehensively before her readers, hoping to prepare the enthusiast to enjoy all the delights of the sport, to encourage the timid, and to assist the inexperienced to define and determine existing limitations. The subject of the care of the bicycle has been carefully treated, some of the means at hand suggested, and the necessary tools and their uses explained. Other topics considered are how the bicycle is propelled, and why it maintains its balance; what the cyclist should learn, how correct form may be attained and faults avoided, and what should be the essential features of the clothing worn.

The author wishes to acknowledge indebtedness to Dr. Legrange, and to Messrs. D. Appleton & Co. for their permission to quote from "Physiology of Bodily Exercise."

Chapter 1

POSSIBILITIES

Bicycling is a modern sport, offering infinite variety and opportunity. As an exercise, at present unparalleled, it accomplishes much with comparatively little expenditure of effort; as a relaxation, it has many desirable features; and its limitless possibilities, its future of usefulness, and the effect of its application to modern economic and social conditions, present a wide field for speculation.

Bicycling possesses many advantages, and is within the reach of nearly all. For the athlete and the sportsman, it opens up new worlds; for the family it solves problems; for the tired and hurried worker, it has many possibilities. The benefits to be derived from the exercise cannot be ever-estimated and the dangers that result from over-doing are correspondingly great; for it is easy to over-exert when exhilarated with exercise and unconscious of fatigue.

It is but recently that the bicycle has become a perfected mechanism, adaptable to general usage, simple and scientific. The railroad makes possible direct and rapid communication between widely separated localities. The usefulness of the bicycle begins where that of the railroad ceases, for it connects and opens districts of country that the railroad has not reached; indeed, it is to the bicycle in connection with the railroads with which the country is gridironed that we must look to make possible the enjoyment of much that is beautiful and valuable, but otherwise inaccessible. To the naturalist, the traveller, and the intelligent observer, cycling offers advantages which are limited only by time and opportunity.

Bicycling has been adapted to serve many purposes; but it is bicycling as an athletic exercise and sport, with the bicycle propelled by human power only, that we shall now consider. The history of the bicycle is modern. The study of its evolution shows the development of a great industry, constantly introducing and applying improvements; most important of these was the pneu-matic tire, which made bicycling universally possible.

Getting under way for even a short cruise awheel has some of the features familiar to the yachtsman. To the skater, the motion is not unlike the rapid, swaying move-ment on the ice, the silence and the rush of succeeding strokes. To the horseman, the dissimilarity of the two modes of locomotion, after the settling to work has been accomplished, is very striking. For the uninitiated and for some others, bicycling does not possess attractions. The bicycle is a familiar object, not compelling a sec-ond thought. One reason for this is that it is not really brought to the intelligent notice of the casual passer. The cyclist, to the stationary observer or the comparatively stationary pedestrian, is such a fleeting instantaneity that, unless thrown among enthusiasts over the sport, few of the unenlightened would be tempted to try it; for they are as unappreciative of what the wheel means to the cyclist as is the countryman, who lives near a railway, of the intricacies of commerce which are indicated by the flying mail.

To the lover of out-door life the bicycle presents a succession of wonderful possibilities. Much has been written of canoe-trips and of the charms of cruising among our inland waters; as charming and as attractive is land travel on the wheel. Bicycling, moreover, combines the best features of many other sports with advantages peculiar to it, for instance, the cyclist must work, and there is much pleasure in watching progress made with so little effort—the work all his own, the machine but a means of locomotion—enjoying and appreciating all the beauties of the country traversed, while yet conscious of the power to hasten away as soon as the surroundings cease to interest or amuse. By the scientist and the naturalist, no encouragement is needed; the bicycle at once compels their attention. The lover of horses may fear that this new mode of locomotion may interfere with his sport—the same objection that was advanced against the introduction of the steam engine. But the bicycle does not displace; it is rather a link in the chain connecting driving and railroading. Bicycling, furthermore, means good roads, not as a luxury, but as a necessity, for it is impossible without them. Rough country may be crossed, but the bicycle must be pushed or carried across it, and this is not practicable for any considerable distance.

The bicycle, though a simple machine, is a complicated mechanism simplified. The principle that keeps it from falling is a well-known one—that of the gyroscope, the only known mechanism that overcomes gravity.

The bicycle has its limits, determined by the powers of its rider and the surface ridden over. The motion is unquestionably fascinating after the control of the machine is acquired; and there is an accompanying exhilaration that is peculiar to the sport, and always something to conquer, something to accomplish, besides the direct benefit to be derived from the exercise.

There is a great variety of methods of bicycling, whether for exercise, transportation or travel. In travelling, the country all about soon becomes, as it were, your own domain. Instead of a few squares, you know several towns; instead of an acquaintance with the country for a few miles about, you can claim familiarity with two or three counties; an all-day expedition is reduced to a matter of a couple of hours; and unless a break-down occurs, you are at all times independent. This absolute freedom of the cyclist can be known only to the initiated, and as proficiency is acquired, it becomes a most attractive feature of the sport.

There is bicycling weather, as there is skating weather, yachting weather, or weather favorable for any out-door sport or exercise. But it is easy to wait for bicycling weather, and nothing has to make way for it. The machine is always ready, and that is all that is needed if a suitable country is accessible. On the road the bicyclist is rendered independent of assistance, for everything needful is prepared for him, and parts and repair supplies can be carried and need but little room. Only inattention or carelessness should cause delay. Still, proper preparation is essential to enjoy bicycling at its best, and the bicyclist should be ready to meet any emergency.

That there is necessarily the element of sociability about cycling is evident. There are so many stops, and the dusty wheelmen grouped among their wheels at the roadside have always the bond of a common interest; from this, transition to individual fads and fancies is easy; there is constant opportunity for acquiring special knowledge and for using it; and almost every accomplishment is appreciated in addition to capability as a bicyclist, and may be utilized in a variety of ways; cheerfulness is an invariable factor; and there is always novelty and the possibility of excitement, for it is unusual, on a bicycle trip, that everything happens as it is expected or has been planned for.

Too much cannot be said of the benefits to be derived from out-door exercise; and one of the best features of bicycling is that it brings so many to enjoy out-door life who would otherwise have little of either fresh air or exercise. Proper oxidation is necessary to perfect health. The great danger that these would-be bicyclists must face is unfamiliarity with exercise, either general or special. Persons accustomed to athletic exercise know how to prepare for and how to resist fatigue, know what practice means and how proficiency may be attained. The bicyclist unaccustomed to athletics has all this to learn, and more; to him, ultimate success means more time given to study and less time to practice. The novice, however, has the advantage that he has nothing to unlearn, and can profit by the experience of others.

To accomplish the best results, the human machine must not be overworked; and to stop work at the right moment is one of the hardest things to learn, and the most important to success. To learn the construction of a bicycle, the particular duties of all the parts and their adjustment, is a matter of memory and observation. To understand the adjustment of the human machine to mechanical environment requires cultivated perception and special knowledge. But the human machine is so independently adaptable, so hard to put out of order, that it may be cared for by intelligent attention to only a few simple laws. Do not wait for danger signals: know how to avoid them.

Bicycling opens a delightful future to all who attempt it intelligently. The inspiration of the enthusiast is invaluable; but it is the practical theorist who is successful.

A bright, sunny morning, fresh and cool; good roads and a dry atmosphere; a beautiful country before you, all your own to see and to enjoy; a properly adjusted wheel awaiting you,—what more delightful than to mount and speed away, the whirr of the wheels, the soft grit of the tire, an occasional chain-clank the only sounds added to the chorus of the morning, as, the pace attained, the road stretches away before you!

CHAPTER 2

WHAT THE
BICYCLE DOES

The bicycle has been evolved—a mechanism, propelled solely by human power, capable of quadrupling the distance traversable by the pedestrian.

The simple, light, and almost universally accepted machine is constructed to stand a strain tremendous in proportion to its weight; for the modern machine weighs only twenty pounds, and it may be lighter, though for some purposes it should be heavier. The bicyclist is virtually mounted on a set of casters, which propels the weight with much greater ease than can be attained in the act of walking. In walking, advantage is taken of the force of gravity by continually falling forward, and simultaneously placing the feet, with a regular motion, one beyond the other, to alternately receive the weight of the body. On the bicycle, the weight is carried and supported, and the wheels reduce friction to a minimum.

The wheel being set in motion, power is applied to overcome inertia, and speed is increased by multiplying the number of the wheel's revolutions; the application of the gyroscope principle assists materially, and the resistance of gravity is overcome in a degree while the wheels are rapidly revolving.

To set a bicycle in motion requires the expenditure of considerable power. A given rate of speed on the level may be maintained by a minimum expenditure of power. Bodies or masses set in motion maintain their velocity undiminished unless other forces intervene. The bicycle in motion is resisted on the level by air pressure and friction, on the roadway by friction, and by the incidental obstacles of the road. On an ascending plane, it must overcome the additional resistance of its own and its rider's weight, which must be lifted constantly; on a descending plane, it must oppose a constantly lessening resistance. All this resistance and lack of resistance means a proportionate stress laid upon the bicycle, the wheels of perfected result of the highest degree of skill. Each part is tested for so many pounds strain or tension or compression, and each strain is accurately figured for each particular part; each part, moreover, must be able to stand so much additional strain, more than it is ever likely to have thrown upon it, though no bicycle is built to withstand the shock of collision under speed. In case of collision, the older, heavy bicycle was not smashed into fragments, as is the modern twenty-pounder. Something would give way, perhaps; it might break in several places. The light modern wheel holds together or is crushed to pieces, though its rider is less likely to suffer serious injury, the lighter construction having less power to do damage than the cumbrous wheel of fifty or sixty pounds weight.

The cost of a well-made bicycle, of perfect workmanship and finish, represents the amount of skilled labor required to construct it rather than the value of the raw material, although, when it is remembered that each part must be tough, hard, strong and elastic, it will be apparent that only the best of material can be used.

Wheels can be made at a very low cost; but such wheels cannot be correctly adjusted and tested without the additional cost of skilled labor. For the production of a perfect bicycle, the machine of tested strength, simplicity of detail, and beauty of finish, the most accurate workmanship as well as the best material is necessary. A machine or a tool should always be the best of its kind, and it pays to take care of it. A bicycle requires as nice and accurate adjustment as a watch, and like a watch, with regular attention afterwards, will run steadily and smoothly. A bicycle, moreover, as much or more than a watch, is individual property, and each individual wants the best.

Our physical powers have been tested in certain directions; in walking, for instance, we know what we can do, how far we can go, how much it is wise to attempt. The bicycle appeals to us as a means of swift locomotion attained without other force than our own powers four or five times multiplied by mechanical processes. The bicycle enables one to do, to prove one's powers; it puts one in conceit with one's self. When one is not a pedestrian, does not care for equestrian pleasures—and, indeed, in the majority of cases, there is little to compel attention to these means of recreation—the bicycle offers the opportunity to find the limit of one's powers in a new field. It supplies, too, a new pleasure—the pleasure of going where one wills, because one wills. The attention has only to be directed, and the wheel, responsive to touch or thought, moves in unison with the rider's will, flitting hither and thither, that he may enjoy the freshness of nature and the ever-changing beauty of clouds and sky, of sunshine and shadow, of meadow and sea, lake and river, mountain and forest.

Riding the wheel, our own powers are revealed to us, a new sense is seemingly created. The unobserving are gradually awakened, and the keen observer is thrilled with quick and rare delight. The system is invigorated, the spirit is refreshed, the mind, freed from care, swept of dusty cobwebs, is filled with new and beautiful impressions. You have conquered a new world, and exultingly you take possession of it.

Travelling by vehicle or by any public conveyance, the sense of individual responsibility is reduced to the minimum; it is indeed no appreciable factor. You pay so much to be taken up and set down, so much for a reasonable amount of safety, comfort, and convenience. Mounted on a wheel, you feel at once the keenest sense of responsibility. You are there to do as you will within reasonable limits; you are continually being called upon to judge and to determine points that before have not needed your consideration, and consequently you become alert, active, quick-sighted, and keenly alive as well to the rights of others as to what is due yourself. You are responsible to yourself for yourself; you are responsible to the public for yourself; and you are responsible to the public for the rights of others. The upholding of laws and ordinances, the general welfare, public health and safety—problems never before, perhaps, called to your attention—come up one by one for consideration. In short, individual duty, recognition of the rights of others, consideration of means for the proper enforcing of laws, all are suggested to the awakening mind of the bicyclist. The bicycle is an educational factor, subtle and far-reaching, creating the desire for progress, the preference for what is better, the striving for the best, broadening the intelligence and intensifying love of home and country. For all that is beautiful is ours—ours to protect and to cherish.

To the many who earnestly wish to be actively at work in the world, the opportunity has come; they need but to come face to face with it to solve this problem of something to conquer, something to achieve.

CHAPTER 3

ON WHEELS IN GENERAL AND BICYCLES IN PARTICULAR

The form of the wheel is very ancient, its construction modern, even recent. Its evolution has been gradual. First came the round stick or roller, placed beneath a weight; then a roller with its central portion shaped and thinned to lessen friction; then two disk-shaped sections of a log, connected by a bar upon which they revolved, replaced the clumsy stick.

Each wheel or disk then began to receive separate attention. There was the wear on the edge or rim to be considered, and it was found that if its surface were protected, the disk would last indefinitely longer. Then it was noticed that the hole in the centre of the disk wore unevenly, and it was reinforced, and the hub began to take form. When the rim was strong and the central portion of the wheel remained intact, the disk was found to be heavier and stronger than it need to be to support the outer portion of the wheel. Some of the useless heavy part was removed, and the disk pierced with holes to make it lighter; then these holes were shaped between the remaining portions, which took the form of pillars or spokes. A pillar would break, and be replaced by a rounded stick; and thus, perhaps, the rude idea took form of constructing a wheel out of several pieces, for the sake of securing economy, durability, and lightness.

A wheel, then, was well constructed, with a large, heavy piece in the centre to stand friction and bear weight, and with the rim made of several pieces, each piece supported on a spoke, and all held together by a band called a tire. In the course of time the hub became heavier, the spokes thinner, the rim stronger and lighter, and the tire narrower. The bar connecting two wheels was made very strong, with smooth ends for the wheels to revolve easily upon. Pins were driven into holes in the projecting ends of the axle, or bar, and later the pins replaced by knobs, or nuts. Then the wheels were brought closer together, and found to run more easily; and the tire, cutting too deep into soft surfaces, was widened. Attention, moreover, was paid to the roadway, very bad places being filled and smoothed.

A wheel is defined as "a circular frame turning on an axle"; an axle as "a shaft or rod, either solid or hollow, on which a wheel is placed." The first bicycle wheels were constructed like carriage wheels, the limit of that method of construction arrived at. The rim was supported on the spokes, which rested on the hub. The minimum definite quantity of material was ascertained, but the wheel was still too heavy and bulky. If the weight of material was lessened, however, it would fall to pieces.

The bicycle wheel of to-day is a compound mechanism constructed on reverse principles. The wheel is made on the principle of suspension, an inverted application of weight and thrust. The hub is hung from the rim, and the axle supported in that way. Each bicycle wheel is really two wheels, graceful in form, with but one rim, and with two hubs, one on either end of a short axle, the spokes being drawn to a common rim, and made stiff enough to carry weight, and elastic enough to withstand shock. The rim or frame is elastic and durable. To this rim many wire spokes are fastened, and the hubs for each wheel are centred and hung from them. The hubs and axle are wider than the rim of the wheel, and the spokes are fastened alternately to either end, thus giving a tangent strain which stiffens the wheel and gives it strength. The tire is a separate construction, possessing several individual features. The only office of the old tire was to protect the rim of the wheel from wear; the pneumatic tire protects the rim, presents a good friction surface, and is enabled by its elasticity to take the shock and jar of the entire bicycle.

In order that the wheel may turn, the axle must be lubricated; otherwise the inside of the hub will become hot, and wear the face of the axle a little rough. The surfaces then cannot pass, but remain fixed and immovable, and the wheel cannot turn. The introduction of a third material of a different consistency between the revolving surfaces prevents their wearing against each other, and the lubricant is rubbed and rubbed again; there is so little of the lubricant that it does not accumulate sufficiently to cause resistance, and the moving surfaces slip smoothly over each other.

The axle of a modern bicycle wheel is compound, and although there are two ends to the axle, there is but one rim to the wheel. The rim carries all the weight distributed from many points at once; the weights resist each other, and give strength and stiffness. The axle really carries double, two wheels with but one rim; and each end of the axle is supported at so many points that it possesses great weight-carrying power in proportion to the weight of material used in its construction. The weight of the frame is supported on the axles of the rear and front wheels. Of its construction it is sufficient to say that the weight is taken up on the thrust principle and that wherever a point of support for the thrust is located, the frame is strengthened to support and resist the thrust.

By a mechanical application of power, the power of the pressure of the foot on the pedal is multiplied, one revolution of the pedal crank causing the rear wheel to revolve a number of times. In the chain gear the mechanical means is a large wheel on the axle to which the pedal cranks are attached, and a smaller wheel on the axle of the rear wheel. There are teeth on both these wheels, the large wheel having the greater number. The band or chain passing over the large sprocket-wheel has links which engage each tooth of the wheel as the chain passes over it, and as that wheel revolves, it pulls the chain over, link by link.

The small wheel is also provided with teeth, and every time the large sprocket-wheel is turned, if only a little way, it pulls the chain link by link, and the chain link by link pulls the rear wheel tooth by tooth. The small sprocket-wheel revolves as the chain pulls it, revolving oftener than the large wheel to keep count with it tooth for tooth. The number of teeth on the sprocket-wheels determines the multiplicity of revolutions of the rear wheel.

The rear wheel revolves very rapidly, in the process becoming virtually a gyroscope; and a gyroscope will maintain the plane in which it revolves unless other forces intervene. The front wheel takes its motion from the friction of the surface over which it is propelled, and after the bicycle is in motion, the forces that are applied to control and direct its movement are friction and resistance. After the cyclist is mounted, there is the added complication of a constantly shifting centre of gravity, caused by change of balance. The steering is effected by changing the direction of the front wheel, the rear wheel being enabled to follow by a slight slipping over the wheeling surface. If the change of direction is too abrupt, the rear wheel will slip enough to lose its hold on the surface, and the weight of the rider will be suddenly shifted from above the point of support (the axle of the rear wheel) to the top of the rim of the wheel, thus becoming a lever with the weight on the end of the long arm, and the bicycle falls over.

As the wheels revolve, there is a constant pull on tire and rim. Just as the chain is pulled over the sprocket-wheels, the tire is pulled by friction over the surface ridden on. If this surface affords the tire no hold, it is impossible for the wheel to advance, as on a muddy surface. The crank may impart a motion to the wheel, but this motion will not enable the wheel to maintain its place; or if, in overcoming the cranks at the dead centre, too much weight is applied to one side of the wheel, the same thing occurs, and the wheel falls over. There are a number of mechanical means for conveying the motion of the foot to the wheel of the bicycle to cause the wheels to revolve.

There are many ways of constructing a frame, and different designs and patterns of fittings for different parts; but the main idea of the bicycle does not change—a fixed wheel to which motion is imparted, and a movable or guiding wheel, independent of the power wheel, and revolving only because the machine is pushed or pulled forward. This second wheel gives stability, and supports the wheel at a movable point.

We have, therefore, a wheel which supports a frame and the weight it carries. The frame is supported on two wheels, one end of the frame taking the weight, and that end supported on one wheel. The second wheel merely supports one end of the frame. If the frame were attached at one end directly and rigidly to the second wheel, the weight carrying wheel would move in the same plane with it. A child's two-wheeled cart will illustrate this. While moving forward in a straight line, the child is safe until one or both of the wheels begin to travel in a rut, when the rigid handle or tongue of the cart resists the guiding power, and the child is pulled or thrown over. If the tongue or frame of the wagon is allowed play, as it is called, say by being held easily in the hand, the pole may be guided. The supported end of the frame of the bicycle corresponds to the pole or tongue of the cart.

Now, the wheel is made to steer in this way: We have the rigid forks, and a wheel to support them. The forks hold the wheel in the same plane as themselves, but the top part of each fork, instead of being fastened immovably to the frame, passes up through a bearing-head prepared for it in the frame. The wheel is supported, but it can now maintain a separate plane, and as the post of the forks changes its direction, it pulls the frame with it as it advances; and so the controlling or steering power is transferred.

The weight-bearing wheel is led and directed; part of its power is transferred by thrust or push to the front wheel, and as the steering wheel is pushed over the surface, it revolves. As it revolves, part of its power is diverted by the movable head, and as the head is held and controlled by the rider, any desired direction may be imparted to the entire machine.

A bicycle may have either a diamond frame or a drop frame. The drop frame is made to facilitate mounting and to permit the adjustment of a woman's dress. The diamond frame possesses great strength, and can be lightened to a wonderful degree without injury to the thrust and strain-bearing quality of its construction.

A form of triangle is made use of to carry the greatest weight and bear the greatest strain. This triangle is supported on the rear wheel, and has part of the frame attached to it to connect it with the steering-wheel. The steering-wheel is provided with handles by which it may be controlled. The weight of the rider is carried over the power wheel, and the propelling power, a lever movement, is imparted by the foot.

From this description an idea may be formed of how and why a bicycle works; but the details of its mechanism are of endless variety of form and pattern, material and workmanship. Each small part, its form, its use, its angles of surface, its every detail indeed, is the product of the work of many minds for many years. And though the bicycle was looked for, and hoped for, and worked for, its general acceptance came suddenly, and came only when it had been built light enough and strong enough and elastic enough to warrant confidence in its universal usage.

Chapter 4

FOR BEGINNERS

Mount and away! How easy it seems. To the novice it is not as easy as it looks, yet everyone, or almost everyone, can learn to ride, though there are different ways of going about it. Unless the beginner is one of those fortunate beings who mount, and as it were, wheel at sight, little need be said about instruction at this stage of proceedings if a bicycle school is within reach. A few suggestions may be desirable, however, even with a competent instructor.

Nothing more quickly exhausts one's strength than the first few minutes with a bicycle. This is due to the fact that many unused muscles are called upon to do unaccustomed work and to work together in new combinations;

and the effort required and the accompanying nervous excitement produce a sudden and apparently unaccountable fatigue. Normal conditions can be restored by resting long enough to allow repair of the wasted tissues. It is well to stop when a little tired, rather than to persist and finish the lesson, even if extra lessons are necessary to make up for lost time. No one can really learn anything when tired, and it is unwise to attempt it. In this matter no one else can judge for you.

What a horrible moment it is when first mounted on a bicycle, a mere machine, a thing quite beyond your control, and unable even to stand by itself. But it is impossible to tell without trying whether or not you can manage a bicycle. Make the experiment, therefore, and find out. Any competent teacher will guarantee success, and after the first five minutes on the bicycle can tell how long it will take you to learn. The time varies with the individual; the period of instruction may last for five minutes or for six months, without counting extra lessons for fancy wheeling.

Don't try to get the better of your wheel. You cannot teach it anything, and there is really much for you to learn.

What to keep in mind when taking your lesson.—
Attend to the bicycle and to nothing else. Don't attempt
to talk, and look well ahead of the machine, certainly not
less than twenty feet. Remember that the bicycle will go
wherever the attention is directed.

In sitting upon the wheel, the spinal column should
maintain the same vertical plane that the rear wheel does,
and should not bend laterally to balance in the usual
manner. A new balance must be acquired, and other muscular combinations than those that are familiarly called
upon. To wheel by rule is the better plan until the natural
balance of the bicyclist is developed. Sit erect and sit still.

The bicycle must be kept from falling by a wiggling
movement of the front wheel, conveyed by means of the
handle-bar. When moving, the rapidly revolving wheels
maintain the vertical plane by rotation, with but little
assistance or correction from the handle-bars.

It is a good plan, while the instructor assists you, to
pedal with one foot at a time, holding the other foot free.
This will enable you to determine the amount of pressure
it is necessary to exert to cause the wheels to revolve.

When both feet are on the pedals, they oppose each
other. The weight should be lifted from the ascending

pedal, or else the descending foot must push the other foot up until that foot is in position to exert a downward pressure. This instruction applies to forward pedaling only; for back pedaling or backing, the movement should be reversed. Practise pushing first with one foot and then with the other, taking the weight off the opposite pedal in each case. At each push of the pedal, a little pull on the handle-bars, pulling with the hand on the same side on which you are pushing with the foot, will keep the wheel from falling. Look well ahead. The bicycle covers the ground very rapidly, and the eye does not at first receive impressions quickly enough to enable you to know where to look and what to look for.

As soon as your teacher will allow it, take the wheel for a little walk. This may seem rather an absurd proceeding, but it will assist you greatly in learning the feel and tendencies of the machine. Lead the bicycle about carefully, holding the handles with both hands and avoiding the revolving pedals. Learn to stand it up, to turn it quickly, and to back it in a limited space.

The machine heretofore has been arranged for you. Now you can begin to think how you would like to have it adjusted. You will, perhaps, find fault with the

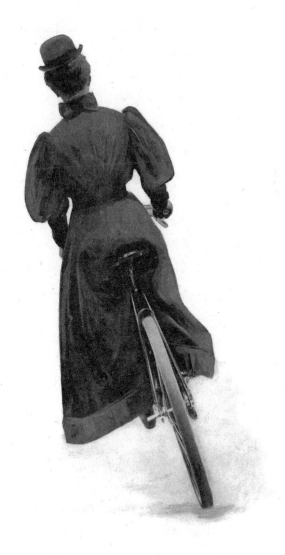

CORRECT POSITION—LEANING WITH THE WHEEL.

saddle. The saddle is a very important adjunct, and much depends upon its proper adjustment. A large, soft saddle is usually preferred by the beginner, and perhaps this is a good kind to learn to balance on; but it is a very poor kind to wheel on, for many reasons.

At first, in practising pedaling, the height of the saddle should permit the hollow of the foot to rest firmly on the pedal when the pedal is lowest. The ball of the foot only should press on the pedal. The foot should be made to follow the pedal as early as possible. Point the toe downward on the last half of the down stroke, and keep pointing it until the pedal is at its lowest, following the pedal with the foot, and pointing downward until the pedal is half way on the up stroke. This carries the crank past the dead centre. To acquire a proper method, attention should be directed to each foot alternately.

To learn to balance, have the saddle raised as high as possible, so that the ball of the foot just touches the pedal at its lowest. Practise wheeling in this way, with an instructor, or alone on a smooth surface where you are sure to be undisturbed.

The hands naturally take a position where it is easy to grasp the handles of the handle-bars. The handle-bar

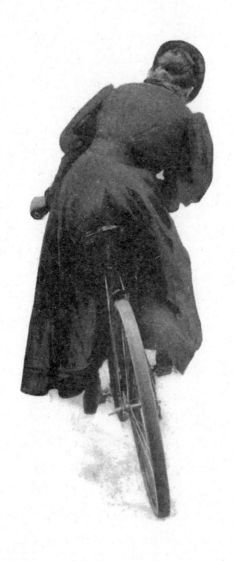

INCORRECT POSITION—LEANING AGAINST THE INCLINATIONS.

conveys two principal movements to the first wheel—a short wiggling movement and a long or steering sweep. The handle-bars also assist in maintaining the seat at first.

The beginner usually exerts too much pressure on the pedals, and has to pull correspondingly hard on the handles to correct the falling tendency of the machine. This is very hard work, and stiff arms and shoulders and blistered hands may be often thus accounted for; they are the result of badly balanced pedaling. To be able to sit comfortably at work, and to feel that it is not so hard after all, is a great advance.

Now, the question of that other foot. By this time which "the other foot" is will have become quite evident; it is always the foot to which attention for the moment is not directed, and which consequently may meet unexpected disaster—a lost pedal, perhaps, with its accompanying inconveniences.

Downward pressure with the foot is easily acquired and needs little effort. To take the pressure off the ascending pedal at the right moment is a more difficult matter. Usually considerable practice in cycling is necessary before the unused lifting muscles are strengthened sufficiently by exercise to permit them to do their work easily.

There is a third movement of the handle-bars—a quick twist in the direction the machine is leaning if about to fall; it is made suddenly, and brings the wheel back to its original position. If the wheel were stationary, and the front wheel were turned, the bicycle would fall in an opposite direction from the front wheel. If the wheel is about to fall, it can be prevented from doing so by throwing the balance the other way by means of the handle-bars. A similar result is accomplished by wiggling the front wheel, and when a bicycle is moving very slowly, a continuous wiggle—changing the balance as the machine inclines from side to side—is necessary to keep it upright.

The body should incline with the rear wheel and maintain the same plane with it, becoming as much as possible a part of the wheel, as though united by a straight bar going from the base of the tire to the top of the head.

The rear wheel and all the weight that it carries is governed by the front wheel and controlled by means of the handle-bars. The rear wheel supporting all the rider's weight, the power is applied to that wheel. The front wheel serves only for balance and steering.

It is not necessary to provide a complete outfit to take the first lesson. If you possess a pair of knickerbockers, so much the better. Wear an old dress, easy shoes and gloves, and a hat that will stay on under any conditions. The clothing should be as loose as possible about the waist. Wear flannels, and no tight bands of any kind or anything elastic. As respiration is increased by the exercise, the clothing should be loose enough to allow of a long deep breath, drawn easily, taken by expanding the chest at the lower ribs to fill the lungs. This precaution being taken, giddiness and short-windedness can result only from over-exercise. Ten or fifteen minutes' practise is enough at first; and a half hour's lesson later, with several stops for rest, is the best rule for many people, particularly those unaccustomed to active exercise.

If you are an equestrian, you will meet with many unexpected problems. The bicycle will do nothing for you, and the lack of horse-sense must be supplied by your own intelligence. It is well, when learning, to remove all bicycle accessories. They are only in the way, and add weight and distract the attention. The propelling of the bicycle—that is the one idea to keep in mind. Make the machine go; shove it along. Never mind if you are not quite comfortable or at ease at first. Sit on your saddle and stay there. Do not try to balance the machine. Lean the way the machine inclines, not away from it, as it will be your first impulse to do. The bicycle is not to be fought against; it is to be propelled and controlled; and the art is not difficult to acquire.

Avoid starting a bicycle on a down grade when you are learning. For on a slight, even an almost imperceptible incline, the cycler must back-pedal; but the beginner wishes to propel the bicycle, and for that purpose must use an altogether different muscular combination.

CHAPTER FIVE

HOW TO MAKE
PROGRESS

You have learned to wheel a bicycle,—have had some lessons, can take the machine and mount it, wheel a little way, and fall off; or can wheel for some time without a dismount, but feel utterly exhausted after a short spin. You have accomplished what you attempted,—you can wheel a bicycle; but you feel dissatisfied. You have tried to ride with friends, perhaps, and have had to give it up; yet you feel that you should be able to do what others have done and are doing all the time. It is very discouraging.

What you should have now is a suitable and comfortable wheeling outfit. You perhaps have a bicycle of your own; if not, a good wheel may be hired reasonably. The matter of dress is now all-important, and a costume suitable for cycling should be selected; it is impossible to do good work or to practise comfortably unless you are properly dressed.

Choose for a practice ride a pleasant day, with little or no wind, and neither too hot nor too cold. The atmospheric conditions are an important factor in bicycling; indeed, beginners are often discouraged by external conditions which really have nothing to do with their mastery of the machine. Take the bicycle out on a smooth road, where you may have two or three miles free from traffic, and as level as possible. If the road is muddy or slippery, wait for the proper conditions. Unless the surface is smooth and dry, it is better to take the bicycle back without attempting to mount it. If two or three miles of good road are not accessible, a quarter-mile stretch or even less will serve. Select a good pathway, however short.

See that the wheel is adjusted to suit you; the saddle of a comfortable height, certainly not too high; the handle-bars convenient to grasp. Assure yourself that all the nuts are secure, the saddle and handle-bars firm. Spin the pedals to see that they revolve easily. Make up your mind before mounting how far you want to go; mount the machine, wheel it for this distance, and dismount. Do not try to look about while wheeling. Give your whole attention to the bicycle and keep your eyes fixed in the direction you are travelling. Avoid hollows and cart-ruts, though these should not occur if the locality for practice is well chosen. If an unexpected hollow or hump should be encountered, hold hard to the handle-bars and press firmly on the pedals, rising at the same time a little from the saddle. The pedals are most important parts, the controlling power being centred in them. If there is a good hand-brake on the bicycle, it is well to note its action and to understand how to apply it; for in case of a lost pedal, its application might give a little confidence. By a "lost pedal" is meant, not that part of the machine is literally lost, but that the foothold is missed on it, and so control of the wheel lost for the moment.

If out of breath, wait until rested. Rest for a few minutes in any case, and look about, and note the surface wheeled over. Then plan another spin, of perhaps a few hundred feet. Fix upon an objective point, wheel to it, and dismount. Rest thoroughly, and mount again. Be careful to avoid becoming chilled while resting, stopping only long enough to restore the natural breathing and to look over the road.

Half an hour of this kind of work at first every suitable day is enough. If you are strong and accustomed to active exercise, the time may be prolonged to an hour or an hour and a half; or you may practise twice daily, morning and afternoon, or afternoon and evening. Cycling weather is an uncertain quantity, and all possible advantages should be taken of it. If tired after the first day's practice, do not attempt to resume it until entirely rested, even if it is necessary to wait for two or three days; for unless the wheel is well understood and the wheeler fairly practised, it is hard work. The practised cyclist controls the bicycle without conscious effort, and may direct his attention to his surroundings; but the novice must concentrate his attention on his machine.

A bicycle should always be handled carefully; for though it is made strong enough for the emergencies of being thrown and pulled and twisted, none of these things improve it. Keep the polish free from scratches, and the more delicate parts free from dents. Do not let the bicycle fall or throw it down carelessly. Learn to balance it against a curb or post or fence or any other convenient object, without injury to the bicycle or to the supporting surface.

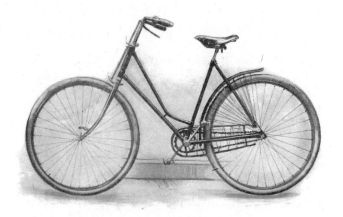

PROPER WAY TO STAND A BICYCLE.

A bicycle will balance in this way: The front wheel kept from moving at either the tire or the centre of the frame; the pedal resting against some firm object.

Do not wheel near anything, but give yourself as much room as possible. A practised cyclist can take a bicycle wherever it is possible to walk, but it is sometimes a feat to do this.

The proper position cannot be too soon acquired. Sit erect and not too far from the handle-bars. Let the hands grasp the handles in an easy, natural position. The saddle should be quite over the pedals to give a natural movement, forward, down, back, and up. The bicycle is sensitive, and yields to almost unconscious direction; but if the eye is not trained to judge distances, steering will be difficult at first. It is necessary to look well ahead, to decide quickly what you will do, and to do it. Pedal fast, but do not hurry. Don't try to find out how fast you can go. This is not a good time for such an experiment; it will be easy later to test your speed. Pedal fast enough to keep the machine running easily and smoothly and to feel it take care of itself a little. It is easier to guide and control it when it is in motion with the wheels rolling rapidly.

It is not a good plan to select a very light wheel for practice. The tendencies and the peculiarities of the bicycle are more readily determined when there is a little weight to resist. Be careful to wear nothing tight, particularly shoes, gloves, waistband, or hat; for they might prove a source of discomfort or even danger.

Learn to steady the bicycle as soon as you can. It will wiggle and wobble from a number of causes. The front wheel must be kept steady. Wobbling results from losing the sense of direction for a moment. To overcome the difficulty, either stop and dismount, or, if it is possible, increase your speed.

Before taking a bicycle out, have any oil that may have settled on the outside of the bearings wiped off, and add a little fresh oil to the oil-cups. The chain or power gear should be lubricated, and any superfluous lubricant carefully removed. The ease with which the bicycle runs depends on proper cleaning and oiling; an illy cared for or badly oiled machine, moreover, is very unpleasant to handle.

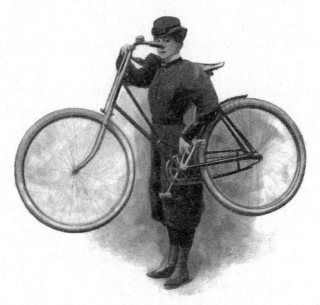

CARRYING THE BICYCLE.

A course of practice will inspire confidence, and wobbling will occur less and less frequently. Then the inequalities of surface will be noticed, and the cyclist will wonder why it is harder to wheel in some places and in certain directions. Parts of the road are covered, the wheeler being almost unconscious of exerting any force, and again in places the foot seems to be pushed up. Ease and comfort in wheeling are dependent to a large degree on the wind and to a much larger degree on the grades and hills. A very little grade, a very slight rise, quite unnoticeable to the pedestrian, is disagreeably obvious to the bicyclist. The difficulty presented may be overcome by pushing on the pedal at the right place as it descends, and at the right time, time and place being also adjusted to the weight and power of the bicyclist. To push at just the right time on a grade assures an easy ascent. Any difficulty in pedaling may be traced to a wrong application of power.

Hill-climbing and grade work require thought and practice. Do not be discouraged because a little bit of a hill seems quite impossible. Overcoming grades is no easy matter, and is usually learned slowly; every time a grade is attempted, however, some progress is made. Wheel as far as it is possible to go comfortably; then dismount, and walk the rest of the way. Never try to mount on an up grade unless you are expert, for this is a difficult and most fatiguing thing to do. When mounting, notice the grade, and if it is downward, do not have the mounting pedal at its full height; and select a clear place to mount in. If an up grade must be wheeled over, it is often advisable to mount in a downward direction, wheel far enough for a start, and then turn to ascend without dismounting. Learn to pedal slowly and steadily and to start and stop easily. These things may be practised at convenient times, and with sufficient practice will be mastered, but meanwhile need keep no one from attempting a moderately long run.

Uncertain attempts at mounting are very fatiguing. Get some one to mount and start you when off for the first long outings; the energy saved can be better utilized in wheeling. Do not be afraid to wheel over small inequalities if their direction is at right angles to the direction of the bicycle; but avoid all ruts and depressions parallel with the wheel's direction. It is easy to slip into them, and difficult to get out of them without a spill.

Never eat a full meal before starting on a bicycle trip; if possible, set the time for starting at least an hour after eating. Ten, twenty, and thirty miles are often covered after the first or second trial. It is better to sit on your wheel and pedal slowly than to dismount. Getting on and off, stopping and starting, are much more fatiguing than wheeling; and it is well to economize your strength at this stage. Always see that the tool-kit is in place on the bicycle, and never go far without a wrench and a screw driver.

The tires also should receive close attention; they should be properly inflated, and the hand-pump carried on a convenient place on the machine. It is never well to use a tire that is not properly inflated. Avoid all broken glass, nails, etc., and do not rest the wheel against a barbed wire fence.

The wheeler who desires to succeed cannot too soon begin to observe and take notes. Early learn to use the wrench yourself, and study how to apply that instrument properly. Study the different parts of the bicycle, and note how they are put together; and particularly observe each nut and screw, and determine its purpose. Each nut must be at its proper tension to hold securely. Study the valves of the tires and learn their construction; and be sure you know how to apply the pump-coupling properly. Learn the names and uses of the different parts of the bicycle, and study their construction. This is mechanical geography, if I may use such a term. Learn to care for your health and how to prepare your system to resist fatigue. Then you will find that you have mastered the subject, and are prepared to avail yourself of the many pleasures of the sport.

The oftener discouraged, the oftener the opportunity to hope again. The art of bicycling is a purely mechanical attainment; and though its complications may at first seem hopeless, sufficient practice will result in final mastery.

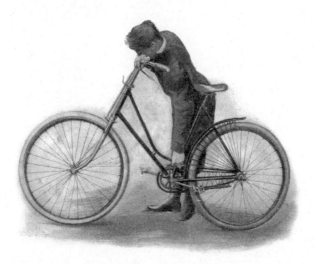

PICKING UP A BICYCLE.

CHAPTER 6

HELPING AND TEACHING;
WHAT TO LEARN

Accuracy is the first principle of cycling; and the would-be bicyclist should learn as early as possible that ease of movement and precision of movement are inseparable; and that bruises and bumps and wrenches, though they may have an educational value, are not a necessary accompaniment of the sport. The skilful instructor need never allow a scratch or a bruise. Some people want to learn everything at once; but only so much should be done at each attempt as can be done accurately, if it be only walking the machine about and standing it up. This exercise is helpful, for walking a bicycle about requires a series of accurate movements, and accurate movement is necessary in learning mounting and propelling.

The bicycle is a marvel of adjustment, and the bicyclist is obliged to adopt movements that correspond with the movements of the bicycle. The more accurate this correspondence of movement, the greater the ease of propulsion.

The lines and angles of the levers of feet and legs must be studied to so apply them as to secure the best results. Avoid undue tension. Learn just how much to lean the bicycle in mounting, just where to place the foot, where to stand in relation to the handle-bars, and where to place the weight on the machine. This understood, mounting is accomplished. The bicycle may be mastered, and easily mastered, by remembering all the things not to do and by doing all the things that should be done.

To assist another to do what you do not know how to do yourself is not an easy task; yet there are people who are willing to undertake it.

A bicycle is so nicely balanced that it is easy to hold it up if it is taken hold of in the right way. Grasp the back of the saddle firmly with one hand, take hold of one of the handles with the other, and the machine is in your power. A person seated on the saddle with a firm hold of the handles of the handle-bar, becomes, as it were, a part of the machine, and when sitting quite still is governed by the same laws of balance that control the bicycle.

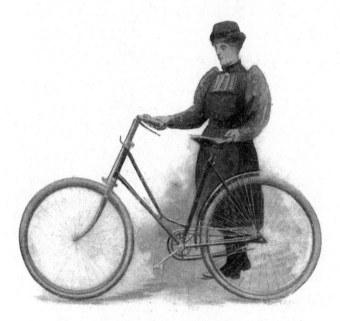

LEADING A BICYCLE ABOUT.

Take hold of a bicycle with some one seated in the saddle, and move it a few inches forward, then a few inches backward, and it becomes at once perceptible that but little force is necessary to overcome the inertia of the combined weights of wheel and rider. The wheel has a tendency to fall to either side, but it is easy to balance the weight on the tires. Then hold the wheel a little toward you, for it is easier and less fatiguing than to hold it from you. If the bicycle is allowed to incline from you, it will pull you over; if it inclines toward you, you can support its weight against the shoulder. If the rider sits still and inclines with the machine, it is easily righted; but if the rider's weight is thrown in a direction opposite to the inclination of the bicycle, the tendency to fall is increased, and the inclined bicycle is pushed over.

Before assisting another person with a bicycle, it is well to note all the tendencies of the machine. This may be done by taking a bicycle and putting it in all the different positions mentioned. The motions are the same whether or not there is any one in the saddle, and it is well to learn to manage the machine without exerting too much force. Stand on the left-hand side of the bicycle, and hold the saddle with the right hand. The steering may be done with the left hand, and the bicycle kept upright by wiggling the front wheel. It is better to do this than to attempt to hold the front wheel still. Walk the bicycle about by the handle-bars only, and you will find that to keep the wheel straight it is necessary to hold the bars stiff, and this is quite a difficult undertaking. Allowed to move gently from side to side, the wheel is more easily controlled.

When assisting a person for the first time, stand beside the machine, see that the pedal farthest from you is raised to its greatest height, and move the bicycle forward until the pedal is commencing its down stroke. Then let the wheeler step in beside the bicycle, in front of you and on the same side of the machine, and grasp both handles firmly. Stand as close as possible to the bicycle, having it inclined toward you at such an inclination that the weight of the wheeler, stepping to the opposite pedal, will right it. Then, while you hold the bicycle still, the wheeler should step on the raised pedal, stand upon the pedal with the knee stiff, and then settle slowly on the saddle; the other foot must find the down pedal. Do not let the machine move yet, but have the beginner go over these movements again, practising them from both sides of the machine until a little confidence is felt.

It is all important to get on the saddle quickly and easily and without necessity for readjustment. If a skirt is worn, it should be arranged before placing the weight on the pedal, and the knee should be slightly bent when the pedal is lowest. The saddle should be the right height; the handle-bars should be a trifle high, that is, when the rider sits erect; the hands should rest easily and comfortably on the hand-grips. Now the thing for the rider to do is to ride and hold on to the handles. Don't let the wheel get away from you. To prevent an accident, should this happen, the beginner should know how to come off the bicycle. An active person can step to the ground before the wheel has time to fall. To get off, step on the pedal that is down, and throw the other foot over.

If the saddle is not right, dismount the wheeler in this way: Have the wheeler's feet firmly placed on both pedals, and see that the down pedal is on the side on which you are standing. Pull the machine a little to that side, and see that the foot is on the down pedal. Then direct the wheeler to step on this down pedal, throwing all the weight on it, and to pass the raised foot over in front of the down foot to the ground. The foot on the down pedal should not be removed until the other foot, placed on the ground, has taken the rider's weight.

Say that you are now going to move, and let the wheeler mount as before. Show that a wiggling movement must be kept up with the front wheel, and say that you will help to do it. See that the wheeler has both handles held firmly, and then grasp the bars just in front of the handle. Keep firm hold of the saddle, and control the balance and push by that, letting the bars do their own work.

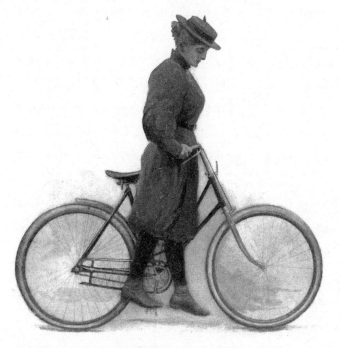

PREPAIRING TO DISMOUNT.

A learner always pushes too hard on the pedals. Take the machine about, and trot it up and down, holding it firmly and keeping it balanced. Should it pull you over, the wheeler can step off without difficulty.

It is much easier for two than for one to help a beginner. A trio of novices can form a very fair school. A bicycle is inclined either to pull or to push, and if supported on both sides, the pulling tendency is avoided and the pushing tendency readily corrected. If ladies are helping one another, the best way is for two to hold the bicycle, standing one on each side of the machine. Both should hold the saddle and both should hold the handle-bars just beyond the handles and above the hands of the wheeler. One should instruct, and the other help to hold the machine.

Let a beginner first learn to mount, then to dismount, practising these movements several times before starting; then, having made sure that the pedal on that side is two-thirds up, come to the left hand side of the wheel, step on the pedal, and be seated in the saddle; then put the weight on the pedal that is down, and step off with the other foot. Repeat several times, mounting from each side, dismounting on the same side and on the opposite side, at command, and repeating. Tilt the wheel as the weight goes on the pedal. Dismount the pupil, and walk the wheel about between you, wiggling the front wheel. Then mount your pupil, and proceed as already explained. After the pupil begins to propel the wheel, very little assistance from the instructor is necessary, and care should be taken not to confuse the pupil as to the amount of work they are doing. Call attention to the ease with which the wheel is brought up when inclined to fall, and explain about turning and steering and wiggling, and what these motions are for. You cannot propel a bicycle unless you know what you are doing; there cannot be guess-work about it. The perfect confidence that comes with familiarity and practice must precede success.

Given three people with one bicycle, all can learn to ride, helping each other in turn. Having learned to mount and dismount, the next thing is to learn to start the bicycle. The weight should be allowed to start the bicycle as soon as the foot, pressing on the pedal as it descends, brings the wheeler to the saddle.

The stop should be learned next. The wheeler should be reminded to notice which is the down pedal, and to step on it with all the weight just as it begins to rise. This will stop the machine, and the dismount is made in the usual way by throwing the other foot over, and stepping with that on the ground. The foot that has stopped the machine should not leave the pedal too soon, but remain on it long enough to control the bicycle.

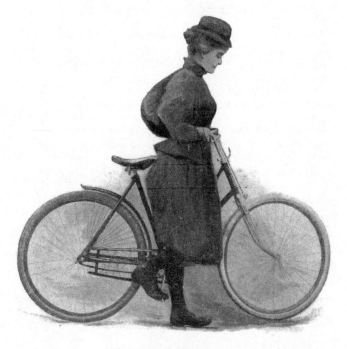

Dismounting.

As soon as the wheeler can pedal a little and has the balance well enough to ride without assistance, the next thing is to learn to ride over ordinary obstructions, and to remain on the wheel for a given number of minutes without dismounting. All this can be taught in an ordinary room or on a piazza; and both teacher and pupil will find a smooth surface, such as a board floor or a pavement, best adapted for the work. Attention cannot too soon be directed to taking the weight off the ascending pedal, and the exercise should not be prolonged for a moment after this becomes a difficult thing to do.

At first the practice leaves the beginner much agitated and breathless; but these conditions are overcome after a few lessons, though experienced riders sometimes experience a return of them when they find mounting difficult and do not notice the grade they are attempting. The sensitiveness of the wheel sometimes puzzles the beginner, and the sense of adjustment is often difficult to acquire.

Nervous work and nervous effort are noticeable in no other sport in the same marked degree. Some seize and adopt its salient points at once and almost unconsciously, but the majority are not so fortunate. The first fifteen minutes on a bicycle are frequently enough to cause thorough exhaustion. The best remedy for this is to take the wheel and walk it about; the pupil should be left alone with it. If fifteen minutes' work is too much, alternate five minutes' work with rest at the next lesson.

The balance and distribution of strength for the pull by the hands is quite important in directing and controlling the machine. The feet are used to propel and to balance. The teacher should note carefully if the beginner errs by incorrect pedaling or by too much pull on the handles, and correct the wrong tendency.

Balance by pedaling comes next in order, and cannot be practised too early; and as by this time a fair amount of speed will have been attained, the natural balance begins to be acquired.

Balanced pedaling and swaying are very different, and should not be confused. The bicycle may be propelled, balanced, and controlled entirely by the pedals; and as this is the best and most important mode of wheeling, it should early be understood and attempted.

The adjustment of the machine should now be taken up, and the wheeler should know how and why the bicycle can be changed to suit individual peculiarities. The wiggling tendency of the front wheel lessens as the wheeler acquires confidence; and its unsteadiness can be overcome and controlled with the balance and by pedaling, with the swaying of the body or the pressure of either foot.

There is much to avoid as well as much to do. Incorrect position means difficult work, almost impossible propulsion and possible personal injury. The knowledge that everything is firmly screwed up about the bicycle, and particularly that the saddle is secure, cannot be too soon acquired. Never attempt to mount or even to try the bicycle unless the saddle is properly secured and immovable. If anything breaks, it is not necessarily your fault; if anything is insecure, blame no one for not attending to something you should yourself have attended to. Always examine the pedals to see that they turn easily; and be sure about that saddle. It is a good deal of trouble to screw the nut up tight for a few minutes, or even for half a minute, but it should be done.

When adjusting the saddle, never be hurried when tools are to be used, for it is necessary to apply them carefully to insure accuracy; and a nut really requires serious attention, for often a good deal depends upon it. If screwed hurriedly, the thread is in danger of being injured, and on that thread the holding power of the nut depends.

When the beginner can balance and propel the bicycle for a little way alone, the really tedious part of learning often begins. At this point beginners become discouraged, for there seems to be nothing new to learn; yet the results attained are unsatisfactory. What is needed is practice.

Practise on a smooth piece of road, with some one running beside the bicycle to give confidence and prevent falls. The proper position in mounting should be studied. In mounting a drop-frame machine, never step over the frame and place the foot on the ground; it is an awkward and ungainly method. Take a proper position, then be sure everything is right, and last of all, step on the pedal, and you are moving.

A good way to practise, if you have no one to help you, is to mount the bicycle in the gutter, and limp along; or if in the country, a roadside fence may give the needed assistance. Grasp a post firmly, and holding by it, try to mount; and study the tendencies and the balance of the bicycle without letting go the post.

Make up your mind how to mount, start the pedal properly, and keep trying until you can ride a little. If a little, why not more? Keep on practising, avoiding faults.

For instruction, the bicycle should be fitted with an instructor's handle, and the pupil provided with a belt having one handle or more. The instruction handle and a hold on the handle-bar are sufficient safeguard for most pupils, but the belt will often give confidence to the timid and aid the instructor.

CHAPTER 7

A FEW THINGS
TO REMEMBER

Two important points for the bicyclist to study are avoidance of road traffic and consideration of the surface ridden over. The law of the road applies to all traffic passing over the road; the law of mechanics to the surface of the road as it affects the bicycle and the cycler. In cities, on much-used thoroughfares, careful work, quick eyes, experience and caution are demanded to insure safety.

The law of the road, "Keep to the right, pass on the left anything going in the same direction," is explicit, and if always observed would render collisions almost impossible. The avoidance of careless and unobservant travellers is quite a study. Passing to the right, you can see and be seen; passing on the left, a traveller moving in the same direction does not become aware of your intention without being notified. You give notice to prevent others from changing their direction and to enable them thus to avoid crowding.

To pass a vehicle on the road, when travelling in the same direction, involves increase of speed if the vehicle in front maintains its pace; should it go slower or stop, and the roadway permits, a change of pace is neither necessary nor desirable, unless you wish to steady your machine. In nearing any vehicle or person coming from the opposite direction, keep your share of the road. Be always alert and observant; do not fail to give ample room to the approaching vehicle; but on the other hand, do not permit yourself to be crowded or inconvenienced, and keep enough of the roadway on your right in reserve in case a change of direction becomes necessary.

The importance of having your machine at all times perfectly under control cannot be over-estimated. Put faith in your pedaling, and never ride at greater speed than you can determine and check at will. Dependence on any brake, however perfect its action, is bad practice.

Vehicles approaching pass each other on the right. In case of collision, the vehicle which has maintained the proper side of the roadway has the advantage in case of legal controversy. In passing a vehicle drawn by horses, the bicycle should keep to the centre of the roadway when possible, leaving the curb for the horse-drawn vehicle. The bicycle can only draw away from the curb, and is limited to one direction. The centre of the roadway, therefore, affords the best opportunity for a change of direction.

Sit well on your saddle, observe the adjustment of the centre of gravity, but ride on the pedals, using the weight as much as possible. Trust to the pedals only for rough riding and for unexpected inequalities of surface. The study of the mechanics of balance, resistance, and friction is most interesting in this connection, as their action affects cycler or wheel or the combined mechanisms.

The law of the road is simple and very generally understood, though there are reckless and ignorant people who disregard it. The law defines where you shall ride, how you shall pass, and sets a limit to increase of speed beyond what is considered compatible with the general safety. There is, besides, the unwritten law of courtesy, more often observed than disregarded; and there is the law you make for yourself.

The traffic of a crowded thoroughfare may be analyzed, and the conduct of a wheel explained and simplified, though travel on such routes is difficult at best and had better be avoided. Given a long, straight road, with two streams of travel from opposite directions. One of these streams will consist of vehicles, quadrupeds, and pedestrians, few maintaining an even rate of progress, fewer still the same rate. The law requires that you pass on the left, and you must await the opportunity to do so. When a clear way opens, take immediate advantage of it, and increase your speed. Should there not be room enough to pass, signal, and the vehicle in advance is bound to make way for you. Should there be a free road to the right, you may take it, but only with the consent of the traveller ahead, and then at your own risk.

Never ride more than two abreast. Riding in single file, with ample room for turning, is better on a crowded street or when making time. For moderate wheeling, the cyclists being disciplined and drilled, the distance between bicycles may be shortened. But control of the wheel should be absolute before this is attempted. When travelling at even a moderate rate of speed, a certain distance between wheels should be observed. When in single file, turn on the same line, but not at the same time as the leader. Inexperienced wheelers are apt to turn at the moment the wheel ahead turns. Should you be following close, keep on your own line, unless you see good cause to change your direction. If the leader wishes to stop, let him turn out: if you are wanted, you will know soon enough. Gain all the distance you can between dismounts. A little drill and the understanding of a few signals will prove very useful.

For the public at large, the bicycle may be specialized to suit individual needs, and locomotion becomes simplified, distances are reduced, and the obliterated landscape of railroad travel takes form and substance. Cycling means travel over well-constructed highways, with telephone and telegraph, post-office and express office, usually easily accessible. To enjoy the full freedom that wheeling should give, little luggage should be carried, yet that little must include all necessaries.

When a party of six or even twelve start to wheel a given distance, what are the problems to be met? All being fairly expert cyclists, in good practice, sociability is incidental while making time. On the road attention, strict attention, to business and to the signals is necessary. Conversation is not prohibited; it is entirely dependent upon the nature of the surface you are travelling.

How to keep together is a vexed question, and a very nice adjustment of animate and inanimate mechanism would be necessary to its satisfactory settlement. The better way is, all knowing the road, to wheel along independently, with an occasional halt, not necessarily a dismount, assembling at intervals of half or three-quarters of an hour. The leader should keep back until the roller of the party is hailed, and has reported, then increase speed again until the next interval has elapsed. Another plan is to wheel with only a given number of minutes headway, this arrangement keeping the roller-up always within hailing distance.

A good leader deserves implicit confidence. He has responsibilities aside from wheeling, for the comfort and convenience of others must be intelligently studied, and consideration for each individual cyclist in the party makes constant demand on the qualities of tact and decision; in other words, the leader must possess good judgment and be as well a thorough bicyclist.

The present rate of wheeling averages ten miles an hour, and greater speed is undesirable, except for special purposes. A point to keep in mind is that every five minutes' halt is a mile lost. The time lost in slowing and stopping should also be carefully taken, as it is of value in reckoning possible mileage.

There are grades to hesitate about, and there are grades to avoid. If a grade seems possible, try it, but dismount the instant it becomes hard work. It is better to dismount too soon than to persist too long. Without regard to the inclination, there are two principal kinds of grades—the increased grade and the decreased grade. In mounting the increased grade, more and more power is required at every stroke to push the machine upward. In mounting the decreased grade, this additional power is not necessary, and the ascent is accomplished with little fatigue. Increase of grade means application of more power in ascending, and an increase of momentum in descending. This is on the whole the most dangerous kind of bicycle travel; for over-work on the ascent, loss of pedals or dangerous coasting on the descent, are to be expected, and danger should be looked for, and observed in time to be avoided.

It is always well to walk an increasing grade, if the hill be long and steep, both in ascending and descending. The decreasing grade has many pleasant features, and on a well-known road may be ridden up or down with ease and with little danger of injury. It is interesting to watch the effect of individual adjustment to hill-work, a group of bicyclists being almost always scattered when mounting a grade.

When and where to apply power and when to make the push tell best on his own machine, each cyclist must determine by practice and experience. Sometimes a long and apparently easy down-grade is rendered dangerous by its increase of pitch; and seemingly easy roads are often difficult to travel on account of an increasing but almost imperceptible ascent. Unless power is applied to the stroke at the right place, much inconvenience from fatigue will be felt, and will soon overcome the ambitious bicyclist.

When short expeditions are to be undertaken—all trips of more than an hour's duration being so classed—remember that lack of preparation means delay, and that ignorance entails discomfort. If the start is to be an early one, go over the bicycle carefully, see that the lamp is in order, that matches are convenient, tools and repair-kit in place, a small envelope of sewing materials with needle and thread and another of red-cross supplies in the pocket.

I have often been laughed at for taking out my lamp for a short afternoon's ride with friends who could ride well enough for their own satisfaction; and as often have I been obliged to help with my lantern's light belated wheels coming in close behind me. A lantern is a convenience at dusk, or even earlier, enabling others to see and avoid you; and this helps more than the uncertain light annoys.

For luncheon on a short trip, it is quite safe to depend on the road; if you carry luncheon, a couple of bread-and-butter sandwiches well wrapped in waterproof paper, and thin slices of cheese in a separate paper, or hard chocolate and water-biscuit, are as good as anything; and such a luncheon may prevent delay in swampy or foggy or damp country from becoming dangerous.

Study the country you are to travel and the road-surface, understand your map, know your route, its general direction, etc. Always observe the road you cover; keep a small note-book, and jot down everything of interest. Use the pocket-compass, even in your home locality, to fix general direction; for when detained at night, such knowledge may prove useful. Fog and rain or a moonless night are bewildering, rendering familiar roads weird and strange; and, unlike the driver or equestrian in the dark, a bicyclist must trust to himself alone. Wheeling in the dark, however, has some advantages, as you are apt to ride in a straight line, and not turn out for bad places in the road; on the other hand, a certain amount of risk is necessarily taken. There should be no close riding, and constant care should be exercised for the avoidance of collision.

Cycling offers endless opportunities for the formation of clubs, and cycling clubs there are of all ages and sizes. A simple form of club for the earlier phases of the sport may be organized in this way: Buy two bicycles, and form as small a club as can manage their purchase. Keep a register, and pass the bicycles from member to member, for say a week at a time, repairs in case of accident to be paid for by the member using the wheel at the time of the accident. The club may later be enlarged by receiving any desired number of members and purchasing additional wheels in proportion. But nothing is so satisfactory as a chosen mount of your own, adjusted to suit your individual needs and kept for your own exclusive use. A bicycle exactly adjusted to your liking should be jealously devoted to your individual use. A beautiful machine should be kept free from fingermarks. Keep a chamois and a clean piece of cheese-cloth at hand where it is kept, and use them. Nickel holds its polish if not attacked by acid or grease. Enamel should be treated differently, with cold water, sponge and chamois, after light dusting.

CHAPTER 8

THE ART OF WHEELING A BICYCLE

There are three very important methods of controlling the bicycle, namely, steering by the hands, guiding by foot-pressure on the pedals, and guiding by the swaying of the body; and these methods may be used separately or in combination.

The wheels are kept in motion either by pedaling, or simply by gravity in descending a grade. The use of the hands on the handle-bar is two-fold for the inexperienced—for steering and for correcting undue pressure on the pedals. The hand opposite the pedal that receives too much pressure corrects the tendency of the bicycle by an extra pull on the handle-bars. This is very good exercise, but it is a useless expenditure of force, and cannot be prolonged without great fatigue. It is the work of hill-climbing done on the level. The feet are on the pedals, and the natural tendency is to press equally at all times on both pedals and pull at the same time on both handles. One pedal must descend, and the other pedal must ascend; they are attached to the same axle, which is turned by either pedal or both pedals. As the pedals are always on opposite sides of a circle, one is always coming up, and its upward tendency is resisted by any pressure, however slight. The lifting of the foot, therefore, from the ascending pedal means easy wheeling. This is one of the hardest things to realize. If there is little or no pressure to resist from the up-coming pedal, it is necessary to expend but little force to propel or push the down pedal; only enough, indeed, to overcome the weight or inertia of the bicycle and the bicyclist and of surface friction, provided there is no grade. But of grades, there are many; and to this is due the infinite variety of the sport of cycling, the muscular development and increased respiration of the cycler.

The handle-bars should at all times be ready to receive a sudden grip or squeeze. Grip the handles hard when you want to hold on, and only pull as much as is absolutely necessary; for if the arms are stiff and rigid from pulling on the bars, they will not be sensitive enough to control the bicycle. The handles of the bar are the ends of a pair of levers; and the nearer the hand to the centre of the bar, the less power is needed to oppose the other hand. When there is a tendency to pull hard on the handles, gradually slip the hands near the middle of the bar, and the pull will ease up. The front wheel, to run easily, should run steadily; and the less wiggle there is, the better for steady travel.

The pedal is the projection on the crank adapted to the use of the foot. There are many varieties of pedals, of differing sorts, weights, patterns, and purposes. The foot placed on the pedal pushes it down; the push is communicated to the wheel to propel the bicycle forward. As the pedal leaves the dead centre, the power begins to take effect, and continues until the dead centre below is reached. Now, it is necessary to push at just the right time and place; if too soon and too hard, the wheels of the bicycle will go too fast, and must be retarded by pressing down on the up-coming pedal. The natural weight pressure of the foot is more than enough to propel the bicycle over ordinary surfaces at a fair rate of speed, without the application of great muscular power.

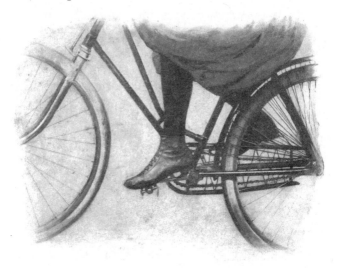

CORRECT PEDALING.

The foot should be placed squarely on the pedal, the ball of the foot only resting on it, and the toe pointing downward. The foot may be made to perform divers duties, and numberless new combinations of pressure can be and are called for and applied.

To apply more power in the stroke, begin to push when the pedal is all the way up, the toe pointing down until at the lowest part of the stroke, ready to follow the pedal around, pushing it backwards, and helping to lift it. Here the toe-clip helps, and holds the foot on the pedal, in the place where the tendency to leave it is greatest. Balanced pedaling is a little different, and weight-pressure on the pedal is used as a factor to overcome the front wheel.

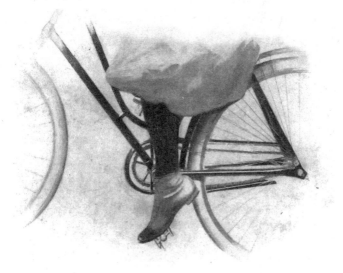

FOLLOWING PEDAL.

Use the weight as much as possible to propel, and reserve the push for hard grade-work. Keep the knees well turned in; it squares the foot and prevents the ankle from receiving hard knocks. When the knee is turned out, the ankle bones are turned in, and so receive many a bruise that could have been avoided. To keep the ankles from interfering, turn the knees in, and ride square leg.

Controlling a bicycle on a down-grade requires pressure on the ascending pedal. Point the heel down or hold the toe up, and an even pressure will be maintained. Let the lift come with the heel well squared and the leg as straight as possible, the weight to be supplied at the right point on the up stroke to control the machine. Always use the weight when possible as a supplementary driving power.

The pedals differ in construction and in material, being differently adapted for racing and for road work. A pedal with a good broad resting surface for the foot is very comfortable, though a "rat-trap" pedal used with a stiff-soled shoe is lighter and preferable. Toe-clips are desirable for those who can use them easily, but for a novice they are dangerous, being liable to cause the mishaps they are intended to prevent. Experienced bicyclers prefer any discomfort to that of a lost pedal, and when wheeling with only a light, even pressure, toe-clips are good reminders; but their principal use is to apply more power and help the foot to carry the pedal around and back.

The swaying of the body controls the bicycle from the saddle. In walking the bicycle about, it is soon perceived that it may be directed by holding the saddle only. The pressure comes from the saddle, and the bicycle is swayed by the rider, by leg pressure against the saddle. There is little or no shoulder movement, and the body, though flexible, does not move perceptibly. When starting a machine, hold it well balanced by the handle-bars, and know how much inclination to allow. Take hold, and mount steadily and easily, and move off quietly, noting the running of the bicycle. Gradually increase the speed, leaning a little forward to lessen any sudden strain and to help the push on the pedals. Then increase the stroke to the desired speed, and the machine will take care of itself. Speed power may be increased, and it is good practice to slow, and start again at will.

Figure wheeling, with a good leader, is capital practice to insure steadiness and increase the power of control over the bicycle. It is not easy to stop suddenly when going at a good rate of speed, and it is well to know your limit of distance in such case; nor is it easy to spring alertly from the saddle when bringing up in a dangerous position, even when frightened into doing it. Back pedal hard, grip with the hands and press down, holding the bicycle still as you reach the ground. The pedals will not get in the way, and it is well to remember not to let go of the machine if you do not want to get hurt. To jump off and hold the bicycle still may at times prevent collisions.

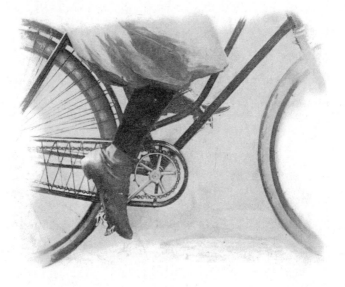

LIFTING.

The cyclist, however sure of his skill, should not throw his machine at any one, even inadvertently. There is much unnecessarily fine riding done—dashing between two passing vehicles, for instance, or rushing through a gap instead of wheeling slowly behind a wagon until an open space is reached; but some prefer the stimulation and excitement of danger to safety, and like to perform such hazardous feats. Steering is a subject for serious consideration; a sharp eye, quick determination, constant care, and a steady hand are needed. A knowledge of steering is essential for safe coasting; and as one of the pleasures of cycling is to descend easily the hill you have climbed, a fair degree of steadiness should be attained. Brakes are important aids. Learn to brake with the foot, but do not resort to this expedient unless compelled to.

Now to consider hill-work. The resistance of the grade is always perceptible; it is not always recognized. As the angle of ascent increases, the powers of the bicyclist are taxed.

The spindle of the pedal describes a circle. The foot part of the pedal revolves around the spindle, and permits the foot to take any angle that is needed for the best application of power, the plane always, however, remaining parallel with the spindle. This arrangement of the pedal allows of ankle-motion within certain limits; and to give greater efficiency, the foot and ankle may move in adjustment with the weight and power to be applied. This is the much-talked-of ankle-motion. The pressure may be applied to the pedal by this ankle-motion at any part or at all parts of the circle that the pedal describes.

As constructed, the pedal permits free ankle and instep movement, prevents cramping of the foot, and allows the foot the same freedom that it has in walking or running. Ease of work depends on proper application of power. To be able to apply just the right amount of push to carry the crank past the dead centre, and to pull it past the lowest dead centre, and to follow the pedal accurately, is the aim of all good pedal work. The push down is almost instinctive; but the lifting of the weight from the ascending pedal can be acquired only by practice, when the muscles have become sufficiently accustomed to the work to move without the effort of mental concentration that they seem to require in the beginning.

The power of the stroke may be given by applying the weight after the dead centre is passed.

The weight should be entirely removed from the ascending pedal, and the balance and sway used to take the pull off the handle-bars by throwing the weight from side to side for that purpose. The weight and balance should be directed in this way: If the push on the down pedal only is used, it must be corrected by a pull on the handle; this pull increases as the grade obstructs the wheel. Skilful hill-work shows in the lessened pull on the handles.

In travelling on the level, the ascending foot is pushed up, and rested by being lifted. There is no reason why the pushing muscles should be stronger than the lifting muscles of the leg except that they are accustomed to do more work.

Always try to ride a hill, but never begin by looking at the top to see how far off it is. Pay no more attention to the surface than is absolutely required by the nature of the surface. Concentrate all thought on the pedals and how best to push or take the pull off the handle-bars. Lean a little forward if necessary, and do not try to increase the stroke. The number of strokes is bound to lessen if the power is not increased proportionately on the ascent. And how can the power be effectively applied unless the work is done intelligently by mental application, or instinctively by the use of accustomed muscles?

Hills should be ridden easily, or not ridden at all. It is easier to wheel up an ascent than to walk up, if the wheeling is properly done. Always stop before the hill proves too much for you. Never think any incline too steep to attempt; this is the first move on the road to successful hill-climbing.

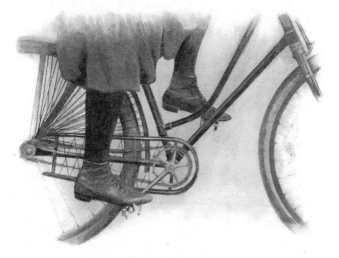

BACK PEDALING.

The seat for hill-work should be made to support the body. The bicyclist should not be obliged to cling to the handles to keep from slipping off over the saddle; there should be something else to push against. To get all possible power out of the levers, there should be a sufficiency of fulcrum for the lever to work against; and the saddle should certainly be made to do duty in hill-work.

If there is no support from the rear of the saddle, the fulcrum must be located at the handle-bars, which should have all possible strain removed from them to lessen the pedal work. A saddle placed at this angle is of little use as a fulcrum on an incline. In all work, levers and fulcrums are kept in position by the hands, unless the weight is supported from the saddle. If this principle of the application of power is considered, the usual difficulty of hill-climbing is overcome. Why should it be harder to wheel up hill than to walk up and push a bicycle?

In the first place, it is necessary to be able to stay on the bicycle without holding yourself on; in the next place, to know how to apply the power; and then to perform the work, keeping all essential points well in mind. Wheel up hill with the mouth shut, or get off; wheel slowly; concentrate power to apply it most effectively.

Power is needed in overcoming both the crank dead centres. The weight should be applied to force the crank downward, and the weight lifted to let the other crank rise. The body sways to ease the handle pull, and the bicycle mounts steadily. The inertia, of course, becomes more apparent as the weight is resisted by gravity; so do not attempt to force or strain, with the idea that hill-climbing is something that must be done. It should be done only when it can be done easily.

The rule for climbing universally recommended reads, "Pay no attention to the hills. Ride them." This is good as far as it goes, but it is of little assistance in mounting an incline.

There are two kinds of grades independent of the angle—the increase grade and the decrease grade, in ascending, and in descending as well; for descending is only the reverse of ascending. In approaching an ascending grade, always note its character, whether long or short, what the pitch is, and particularly if the angle of ascent increases or decreases at the top of the incline, and prepare for the work before you.

Each hill has its peculiarities, which must be studied and conquered. The actual mounting to the top is not all you have to do; you should mount in proper trim, arriving at the summit fresh and fit. It is most saddening to see some one else mount a hill easily, leaving you, puffing and pushing, half way up, and to know that, when you reach the top, speechless and exhausted, that exasperating person will be seated there, cool, contemplative, and comfortable.

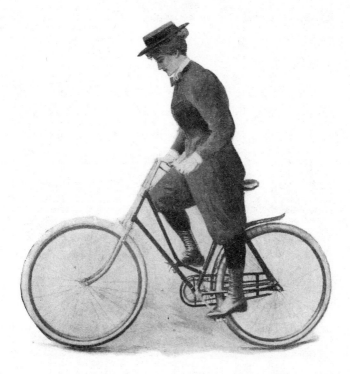

BACK PEDALING—SHOWING DISTRIBUTION OF WEIGHT.

Intelligent practice, however, should result in scientific attainment. The saddle should be adjusted in relation to the pedals for the carrying of the cranks past the dead centre. The angle of the saddle should be studied, and the adjustment permit of its use as a fulcrum in hillwork, while admitting of balance-work on a level and of comfort and ease in coasting. It should support the weight when the feet are on the forks, not merely permit of balancing.

In studying this adjustment, weight, length of limb, strength, and the work to be done should all be taken into consideration. The rule that what is lost in speed is gained in power should comfort the hill climber when, half-way up a grade, the bicycle gradually loses speed, and seems to be stopping, in spite of all efforts to the contrary.

In mounting, the machine is started by the placing of the weight on the pedal, and in hill-climbing the weight should be used to force the pedal down and around. The bringing of the pedal into position where the weight will take effect is the true secret of success. Follow this by making the weight carry as far as possible, prolonging its usefulness by pushing the pedal back past the lowest dead centre, and following and lifting it. But it is useless to prolong the work if the commencement of the stroke is not executed in an effective manner.

The up-coming pedal must either be pulled up, or have all weight removed to permit the power to be fully effective on the down pedal. What is the point where power applied will begin to tell? If the upper dead centre is left to be overcome by the downward stroke of the foot on the pedal, the foot on the ascending pedal is doing no work, only kept from doing harm, held in a cramped position.

After carrying the crank past the lower dead centre, the weight is removed and the angle of the foot changed from pointing the toe down to holding the toe up and dropping the heel. As the foot-rest will follow the sole of the foot, it is a simple matter to change the pressure from pushing and pulling up to pressing and shoving over. Before the crank has arrived at the top of the circle, say at sixty degrees, the heel should be lowered, and the attention directed to pushing the cranks over and past the dead centre. As the top of the circle is reached, the foot levels, and prepares to point the toe to make an effective downward thrust. Rise from the saddle a little at this point, to make the weight more effective, and prepare to carry the pedal back as far as possible. This method leaves very little time for the foot to change its angle. From the toe pointing downward to the toe held up ready to push, the change from pull to push is abrupt, and hill-work depends on correct ankle-motion more than anything else. The ankle-motion may be corrected by swaying, the hands meanwhile being held lightly on the handle-bars ready for emergencies, but not used for the work of climbing.

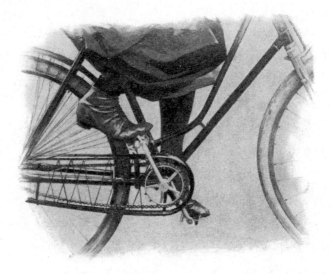

HILL CLIMBING—PUSHING CRANK OVER.

The breathless condition induced by extra work may be remedied; for the upper chest is forced to expand, while, if the arms are held rigid, a plentiful supply of air for the lungs is not insured. (See Chapter on Exercises). Free combustion is needed for the extra power exerted.

The bicycle and its load are lifted, and a given weight requires a given power to lift it. That power must be supplied by the stored force of the human body, and must be utilized to the best advantage if the work is to be prolonged. Hill-work is not impossible of achievement; but it requires intelligent work unless one applies mechanical laws intuitively. Easy hill-work is delightful; it is work, hard work, but work done without strain. Nothing, on the other hand, can be more injurious than forced hill-climbing; the strain on heart and lungs is severe, particularly for one wearing a tight belt, or any constrictive clothing about the waist.

Because a hill looks rough and the surface difficult, it does not at all follow that it will be bad wheeling. If the tires are not too full, inequalities of surface are an assistance, helping to block the wheels, and preventing them from slipping back, while the soft tire takes up the stones and bumps, holding on by them. Always look well at your hill on approaching it; study its inclination, determine its grade, and the nature of its surface, and quickly decide how best to attack it.

On mounting the top of a grade, never hurry or increase speed; wheel along slowly and easily, with the mouth shut, until rested and really ready to start up. If there is a good coast, don't hurry to it, but keep working gently until the balance of the respiratory organs is fully restored. Then take the coast, and all the benefits of hard work, and rest, and the exhilarating effects of swift motion and free oxidation are fully realized.

To work in balance or equilibrium is the aim of hill-work, and there should not be too abrupt a transition after severe exertion. Pedal along at a pace to restore the breathing after hard work, then change; never dismount when breathless, but wheel along slowly. The strain is thus much less than by forcing the body to accommodate itself to a change of position just when a general easing is required, a general slackening of all the muscles that have been at work.

Rest always before dismounting long enough at least to restore breathing; and rather than coast after climbing, back-pedal gently and slowly if the grade should descend from the top of the ascent.

Never let a hill get the better of you, if it is one that you have a chance to attack a second time. Set to work and study it. Find out the changes of grade, and prepare for a change in the amount of power at the proper place in the incline. See if the grade is simple, prolonged, or compound. If the surface is very smooth, it will be more difficult. There is a bit of road that I remember well, a country road, seemingly good enough, with a little grade perhaps in some places; but, one after another, it dismounted us all. A heavy Telford pavement was laid, but there was still a mile and a half of that road that winded the best of us every time. Though it was up grade all the way, experience had taught us that at places we must stop, and mount again and go on. Our machines were heavy, but this fact did not explain what puzzled us; for it ought not to be easier to start a heavy wheel up a grade than to continue to wheel up steadily. Knowing this bit of road so well, we were on the lookout to note its effect on others; and there were always wheels lined up at some part of the road, and a curious variety of expressions on the countenances of their riders—puzzled defeat on those unacquainted with the road, and sad determination on those who knew it too well.

After a careful study of this grade, that was long but not steep, and seemingly not difficult, we found it made up of a series of differently inclined planes and curves, the up-curves all against us; and, taken from foot to top, there was a continued increase of pitch, with certain changes that were all against wheeling; and moreover a generally increasing pitch for the whole distance, and four places of change of grade, each change an increase of pitch and an increased angle of ascent. The smooth surface concealed these difficulties at first, making the deceptive stretch appear easy and inviting. It was like the inside of a curved line set with scallops.

To overcome this most difficult kind of incline, wheel along at a good pace, note the increase of grade, and drop the heel at the beginning of the down stroke, or rather while the pedal is half way on the up stroke and the foot is prepared to resist the change. Take into consideration the fact that an increase of power is necessary; look where to apply it, adjust the balance of the body to the work, and your work will be effective.

CHAPTER 9

POSITION AND POWER

The racing wheelman has adopted a position that has received much censure—a position accepted as the one enabling applied power to produce the greatest speed. If this position is analyzed and compared with the erect position, several interesting features may be noted, and by comparing the two positions, important information may be gathered.

The bicyclist seated upon the saddle, not against it, has little power for work. The thrust is downward; there can be no forward push or backward thrust, unless the hands grip the handle-bars and pull against the push, if the push needed is greater than can be resisted by the weight of the body.

The power of the stroke is all in the downward direction; there can be but little power in the forward thrust; the most important part of the stroke in hill-climbing is that given by getting behind the pedal and pushing it down. If the saddle be too far forward, power is again lost in the push and thrust, and the up-and-down motion must do the work, and power is lost on the down thrust, though added in the upward and backward push.

We may conclude that a proper position has much to do with the work of bicycling; that there is more than one correct position, different positions being adapted to different work. The racing position on the bicycle is the position for speed, and is the position of the running athlete. It is not adapted to moving at a moderate pace or to being maintained for any length of time. It is the position in which power may be most readily converted into speed; where the leverage may be applied with the greatest efficiency, and the greatest amount of work accomplished in the least possible time.

The drop position also takes the strain off the upper leg muscles, and is desirable on that account, apart from the fact that more power may be exerted from that position. The leg does not straighten out, and is always ready to give a powerful stroke and maintain an increased or even speed. It is a position of continuous movement; and if the weight and all the muscles are not directed to propel, the weight is improperly supported on all fours.

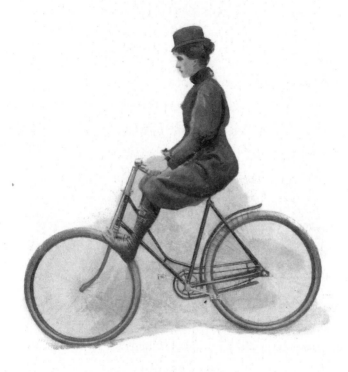

COASTING.

The position for speed where the weight is distributed between handle-bar, saddle, and pedals is not suitable for road work, nor can it be maintained for any long period without injurious results. It is the position where power is best converted into speed.

For prolonged work a different position is demanded. Here speed is not a necessary factor, but ease of movement and continuous movement are essential. We are not anxious to convert power quickly, but rather to reserve our powers, and use them slowly.

For pleasure riding and ordinary exercise, the erect position is the best. The drop position is the racing or running position; the erect position, the position of ease.

Here the saddle question presents itself. The saddle should support the weight while seated, or, in the racing position, hold the weight; it should not hamper movement, and should be comfortable for coasting. In moving over the ground, the relative position for the balance of the cyclist changes according to the grades; and the seat should be adjusted so as to be adaptable to the different positions required to enable the bicyclist to change the balance for the work of the moment.

There is also the position adapted to quick work and exercise. Change in adjustment of the application of power varies with the amount of work done by the bicyclist in covering a certain distance. The resistance caused by change of speed and varied wind resistance have also to be taken into the calculation. People of different lengths of leverage must study the different adjustments of the machine to produce the best results for the different kinds of work required of the machine.

When a hill is to be surmounted, the climb should be made without effort, that is, effort understood in its technical sense. The position should be such as to permit of work being done by the foot, and the power should be applied at the right time and place. Assistance by a pull on the handle-bars means lessened power on the stroke. Effort succeeds effort. The work should be done by the foot, the pelvis being the fulcrum. The saddle should be the real fulcrum. If the hands are used to do the work by pulling, the pelvis becomes the only fulcrum, and the bicycle saddle is not used at all for the application of power. The weight should be made to do as much of the work as possible, and the added resistance of lever pressure made auxiliary.

To obtain leverage for the hands, it is necessary to use a fulcrum. Where is that fulcrum located? Each set of muscles pulls on its point of application—the hand on the arm, the arm on the shoulder, the shoulder on the thorax, the thorax on the pelvis. If more power is needed, it must require effort.

In hill-climbing, effort is a physiological phenomenon associated with great expenditure of force. In making an effort, exerting force, the air-passages of the lungs are closed, the air in them making of them an air-cushion, as it were, which acts as a fulcrum for certain extra muscular combinations. This accounts for the feeling of suffocation experienced in severe hill-climbing, which should never be prolonged. The hill should be climbed with the hands held easily, not gripping the handles; and gripping and pulling on the handles, it should be remembered, lessen the power for prolonged work. Squeezing the handle-bars induces involuntary lung compression, and pulling on them adds to the strain. Lean forward, if need be, to balance and maintain the equilibrium, but do not maintain the centre of gravity by pulling on the handles.

The fixed position of the arms, when sitting with spinal column erect, certainly prevents a full, free inflation of the lungs; the shoulders are held fixed, and between the saddle and the fixed shoulders there is no up and down lung-play. In running, the forearms and shoulders permit free chest expansion. In the racing position on a bicycle, the arms and shoulders take the same relative position as in running, and a full, free lung expansion is obtained.

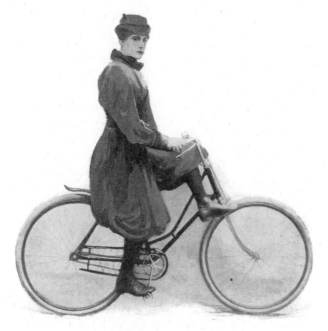

WHEELING ONE FOOT OVER.

No rigidity is maintained between shoulders and saddle in the racing drop-position.

For speeding and work of that kind, the position that

allows of the greatest flexibility as well as the greatest leverage is the position to be chosen.

In travelling and in every-day wheeling, the position should be one permitting the minimum expenditure of power; the weight should be supported, yet the position should be such as to permit the weight to be used as a propelling power. The hands should be held where they are supported and in the position where they can most easily control the wheel under any change of conditions. The saddle should be placed where the foot can act most effectively at all parts or at as many parts as possible of the circle that the pedal describes. The height of the saddle should be calculated to permit of extension of the leg without supporting the weight on the saddle, which causes compression of the larger veins and arteries. The foot should at all times be fully on the pedal; that is, the position should permit of throwing all the weight on to the pedals, whatever the position of the cranks at the moment. The handle-bar should be adjusted; also length of arm and relative position; and the weight, height, and curve of bar adapted to suit individual build.

Length of crank, gear, height, position, and adjustments of saddle may be used as factors in adjustment of position for ease of movement and prevention of fatigue. Each individual has different combinations of lever power, varying with the lengths of the different parts of different limbs. One may have a long thigh-bone with short lower leg; another may have just the reverse combination—short thigh-bone and long lower leg.

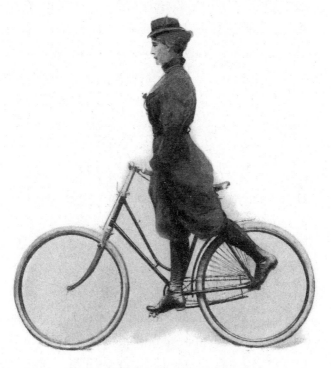

WHEELING FROM THE PEG—SHOWING
DISTRIBUTION OF WEIGHT.

The crank is the lever of application of power; the gear, the power in resistance. The gear determines, in a sense, how much force is needed; the length of crank, combined with the levers of foot and leg, the proper or most comfortable lever for overcoming that resistance. Long-limbed people do well on long cranks, short-limbed people on short cranks,—the question of length of limb to be determined, not by actual measurement, but as to the proportions in weight and length of limbs generally. Either too long or too short a crank will produce numbness and fatigue. The leg and foot on the crank as it works form a crank lever movement. The crank of a bicycle should be of such length as to permit of the greatest amount of force being conveyed along the lever movement with the least resistance.

The sprocket-wheel is the weight to be moved by the crank; but the crank is only one of a series of levers.

The knee, the ankle, and the pedal-pin must revolve in a circle or a part of a circle; and each individual must find out the size of circle that is determined by the crank that will best move in adjustment with his individual lever combination. A small circle on the pedal may mean cramped or uncomfortable movement for a long-limbed cyclist; or a large pedal circle too great distance to traverse on the stroke for a short-limbed cyclist. A stout person working on a high gear, with a crank adapted to his requirements, makes fewer strokes of the pedal for distance traversed, but expends more power at each stroke; therefore, when wishing to reduce weight, he should use a low gear, working rapidly, and when wishing to travel easily, a higher gear. A thin person should be careful to choose such a length of crank and such a gear as will give ease, so that undue fatigue may be avoided.

The position of the saddle should be most carefully considered. It should be just far enough back to permit of getting a forward pressure on the pedal against the crank, as it were, at the top of the stroke, and yet have something to work against in hill-climbing. The tilt or inclination should be studied as well as the build of the saddle; its height from the pedal should allow the foot, when on the pedal, at its most distant point from the saddle, to press with the ball firmly on the pedal; and yet the saddle, when the leg is extended, should not press so as to compress the large blood vessels of the inside of the leg as it rests against the saddle.

The handle-bar adjustment permits of individual preference to a certain extent. The handles should be within easy reach of the hands and below the line of the elbow. If above the level, power is lost, and the controlling sense of direction as well. The grip on the handles is instinctive, and as there is much work for the hands to do, they should be able to grip easily and quickly, and to move easily in all directions that the handles take, retaining their controlling power undiminished. A position with the hands reaching down a little gives more power than a position with the hands reaching up; and in this position the leverage of the elbows and the power of the shoulder and upper arm may be more effectively exerted.

Speed work should be done only on a track or a place set apart for that kind of work; and the most delicate adjustment and balance of weight and pressure should be studied to produce the proper results. Scorching, also, to be effective, should be done only on a track, and the position for the work should be planned most carefully. High speed over rough surfaces on even well-made roads may prove disastrous if the position for the work is not a correct one. Serious injury may result to the bicyclist working incorrectly, with wheel out of adjustment.

Scorching and racing, however, are not properly part of the subject of bicycling, but are a sport, and should be separately considered.

The adjustment of position may be changed for rest or for any particular purpose; but for practical purposes it is well to adopt a fixed adjustment of handle-bar and saddle and length of crank and gear, and adhere to that, endeavoring to acquire the best form on a machine adapted to suit your individual requirements.

A bicycle should be used only by the person for whom it has been adjusted; for comfort on a bicycle depends on such infinitely small adjustments. Never lend a bicycle or a tool, and never make any change in adjustment by guess. For ordinary use, the saddle should be a little back of the pedals and not too high, and the handles within easy reach. This will allow of the balance and adjustment of weight and balance to suit changing conditions of surface and grade.

Sprinting is often tempting, and comparatively harmless. Scorching is a form of bicycle intoxication, and the taste once acquired, the bicyclist craves its excitement, caring little for the other pleasures of the sport. The scorcher sees little, hears little, and is conscious of little but the exhilaration of the moment, and seems to be imbued with the idea of consuming a certain amount of tissue in a given time. Scorching is a form of bicycling hardly to be commended, and reckless scorching is to be condemned at all times. Sprinting consumes a large quantity of material in a limited time, and though it is well at times to practise speeding, still the getting up of speed involves considerable expenditure of power and greatly increased momentum, and should be indulged in only by those who understand the limit of their powers and know what they hold in reserve.

The wheel of to-day was evolved on the race-track and for the conditions determined thereon; and the amateur bicyclist owes much to the professional wheelman. Improvements in construction, in detail, and in adaptability have reached a certain limit, a limit of possibilities in certain directions. It behooves us now to accept the machine and to adapt ourselves to its requirements and to avail ourselves of all that it offers.

The elasticity of the machine, the resiliency of the tire, rigidity of frame, position, vibration, and concussion should be next considered.

On a bicycle fitted with a rigid saddle and with hard tires, well blown up, the vibration that is conveyed through the entire machine is very perceptible, even on a smooth wheeling surface. Over uneven country, Belgian blocks, or other rough or corrugated surfaces, the vibration produces concussion; and if too erect and rigid a position is maintained, fatigue, if nothing worse, is sure to result.

On a horse the position, while erect, is studied to lessen the concussion; the weight is carried well under to avoid it. The flexible curve of the spine is there, though not perceptible, as the body is held erect and in balance. The lower part of the body becomes part of the saddle, the upper body flexible from above the hips. The concussion comes as each of the horse's feet is placed on the ground; while concussion on the bicycle is produced by the change caused by each inequality of surface. The pneumatic tire lessens this to a degree, if not blown up too hard; for inequalities sink into the yielding surface that would make a wheel with a hard tire bump.

The frame should be stiff to hold its direction, and the saddle elastic enough to interrupt the vibration of the frame. The position on the saddle should be studied to prevent tension or compression of any of the joints, large or small; and the spine should be easily erect, not stiff and rigid, but flexible.

The sense of balance and the adjustment required to balance the bicycle tends to keep the body flexible. The danger to be avoided is concussion induced by a rigid position—a position where, the bones being held closely against each other by tense muscles, shock is easily conveyed over the entire body.

Let the weight come well on the saddle, in such a position that it can be shifted to the pedals at will; and let the whole trunk be flexible, elastically flexible, equally in all directions. Then the bicycle may be controlled almost unconsciously and from the saddle, the hands being used only in an auxiliary manner. The front wheel may be steered and controlled from the saddle by means of the power over the front wheel gained by the bicycle frame construction.

Bicycling can be thoroughly enjoyed only when the machinery ceases to require constant and concentrated attention. The rhythmical movements of a bicyclist at ease, master of the conditions, comes only with confidence and the persistent practice which causes all the muscles to move easily together in uninterrupted combinations, and the bicycle no longer to require conscious attention.

CHAPTER 10

DIFFICULTIES TO OVERCOME

There is the mounting difficulty and the steering difficulty and the pedaling difficulty; and then there is the general difficulty of doing all these things together.

The first thing to do after learning the theory of starting and stopping the machine is to make it go. No matter what happens, keep it going, the faster the better, until a taste is acquired for the pastime; until the going-forward-forever idea seems to have taken possession of you.

Then you want to try it again, but mounting seems more difficult than ever. The machine will not do anything it ought to do; it bucks and kicks and stops and spills and slips, and will not stand still, or even move on.

You know how to mount, or think you know; but that knowledge does not seem to aid materially in overcoming the tendencies of the machine.

Now be sure that you do know what to do. The first thing to know is that the weight placed on the pedal starts the machine; that the foot on the ground will hold the machine, and keep it from starting; that the machine when in motion will move without falling, and when at rest will not stand still unless held up.

Then determine the amount of inclination the bicycle requires to balance against your weight. The weight placed on the pedal pulls the machine up to a vertical plane; and the inclination to be calculated for soon becomes an accepted quantity. In gripping the handles and inclining the machine, the balance that is felt will set you up on your wheel.

In mounting, the beginner is apt to stand too far behind the mounting pedal. The position should be beside it, and the mounting foot be placed over the frame and on the pedal. Then, raising the weight by means of the handles, step off the ground, letting the pedal take the weight. Do not give any push from the foot on the ground, but step off the ground as you step on the pedal.

Stepping on the pedal sets the machine in motion, and rights it at the same time. There is nothing now to do but to let the pedal lower you to the saddle, and hold the other foot up until the other pedal comes around and carries the foot forward.

In mounting, the weight should be distributed between the handles and the pedal until seated on the saddle. To practise mounting, take the wheel, and start on a very slight down grade. Never attempt to practise mounting against a grade, no matter how slight the inclination. A careful instructor teaches mounting and dismounting thoroughly; but if a poor method has been acquired, practise alone until you have gained confidence and perhaps a few bruises. The only way to succeed is to try and try again. Practise fifteen minutes at a time, for it is fatiguing work; and do not become discouraged. With sufficient practice, the difficulty vanishes.

Never practise mounting when tired; for you should be alert, and all your muscles responsive. But persist; practise first mounting, and then dismounting; and then rest by walking the machine about to learn its balance.

Any one who rides or drives, or rows or sails, knows something of the art of steering,—pulling or pushing on one side or the other to change direction,—and on mounting a bicycle has only to apply knowledge already acquired. In steering a bicycle, look directly over the centre of the handle-bars in the direction you wish to take, and push or pull the wheel until the centre of the bars coincides with your objective point. This is really what is done; but the machine is so delicately sensitive that you change its direction almost without knowing that you are doing so. You go where you look; the hands follow the eye; and the art of steering a bicycle resolves itself into knowing where you want to go, and looking in that direction as you move. In steering or mounting, always have an objective point. Look up the road well ahead, and keep the general direction.

A difficulty early experienced is uncertain steering and an uncertain sense of direction. When you are out for practice, look well ahead towards the end of your road over the handles. Novices run into anything they look at, and must concentrate their attention, therefore, on the direction the bicycle ought to take.

The weight inclined from side to side steers the bicycle; pressure on either pedal steers it as well.

Correct and effective pedaling is a very difficult

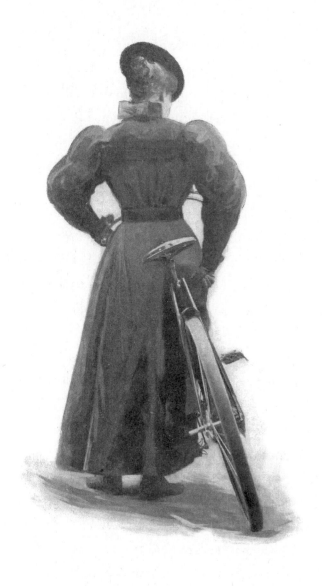

PREPARING TO MOUNT—SHOWING INCLINATION.

attainment, to be acquired only with care and practice. First make the bicycle go, then study how you do it, and improve your method. Keep in mind the points that are required for correct pedaling. The early difficulty experienced is to keep the knees and ankles in proper line. Turning the knees in and the heels out will prevent the ankle-bones from striking, a difficulty that many experience.

The reason that mounting is so difficult for some is because the foot is placed incorrectly on the pedal, with the toe pointing out. The foot should be parallel with the frame of the bicycle, and the knee turned in; or else, when the weight is raised, the ankle will strike, and the discomfort of the blow will render the attempt to mount unsuccessful. The position seems awkward until correctly acquired; but the awkwardness is due usually to lack of confidence to come close to the machine and to taking a position too far back of the mounting pedal.

The change of direction on mounting often proves confusing, and the bicycle must be steadied, and made to keep its direction at the same time.

Choose your direction, and assure yourself of plenty of room to work in, away from trees or stones or other

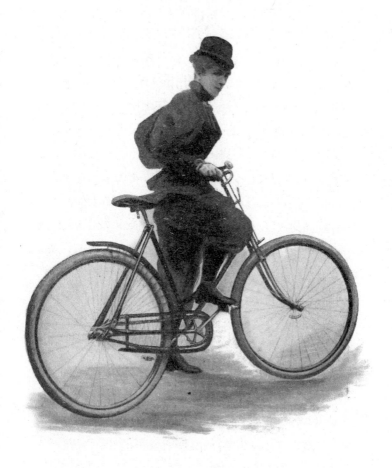

INCORRECT MOUNTING POSITION.

objects that might prove a source of danger in case of collision. Then mount and go. Keep these two ideas well in mind. If you are uncomfortable, stop and get off; don't try to adjust anything while in motion. When you get on, go. You cannot get on and keep still. Do not get on unless you are ready to go; keep going when you are on; and the mounting difficulty vanishes.

Steer steadily, and be quick without haste. A hurried change of direction can only be made without danger of a spill by an expert, and then only in an emergency or for track-work. Bicycling requires precision, and haste or hurry is out of place, while quick and alert movement is required.

Take the bicycle out and do as much as you can with it. Part of the fun is conquering difficulties, and each difficulty overcome is an achievement.

Another difficulty experienced is striking the saddle in mounting. This is usually due to springing from the ground to the saddle, or attempting to do so, instead of stepping on the mounting pedal, and supporting and holding the weight on the handle-bars. Of course, if the weight is not supported on the machine, and the machine is started, it cannot carry the weight forward. The saddle will strike, and push you over. Mount by means of the handle-bars; let them take you; shift the weight up by them on to the pedal. Then lower the weight to the saddle, step clear of the ground, and lean a little over the bars if necessary to clear the saddle.

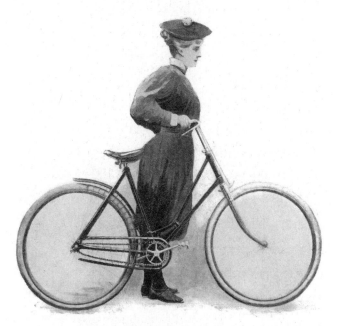

MOUNTING—PREPARATORY POSITION.

In mounting a bicycle, you mount up on the pedal, and settle from that down to the saddle. If the pedal strikes the other foot, it is because the foot is not held up. Do not be in dread of that other foot; hold it well up out of the way, using the mounting foot to make the machine go.

Too great inclination of the machine will spoil the mount, and insufficient inclination will have the same effect. The front wheel must be held in line with the frame, and any wrong tendency corrected by the handlebars after the weight is raised on the pedal, and the machine is upright.

Many good tires are ruined by ineffectual efforts to mount. The machine is pulled against the tire, and it is hard to understand why the tires are not torn off or ripped to pieces. The light wheels are not made to stand such usage; and it is a mistake to subject a new wheel to it. The rubber is pulled sideways (a proper way to pull a tire off), and the novice is fortunate if the bicycle is not all pulled out of true by being strained in directions not calculated to resist wear and strain. A twenty-pound wheel may be pulled out of true and so bent and untwisted by ineffectual mounting efforts that it cannot be restored without labor that amounts to practically rebuilding the bicycle.

In turning a bicycle, always lean in the direction the machine is inclined. Lean in the direction you want to go, and very little correction will be needed from the handle-bars. In turning, lean with the wheel, and meet it with the handle-bars. Meeting the machine is done continually, and is done by swinging the front wheel to meet the inclination of the bicycle on whichever side it has a tendency to fall. Bringing up is done by pulling the wheel around a little further quickly, and very quickly back again. The frame is lifted by the front wheel. This is explained in the principles of bicycle construction. When an obstacle, as a car track or rut in the road, is met, the obstacle must be crossed squarely; or if obliged to make a different angle, the angle should be met with the front wheel at the instant of contact, and a proper balance maintained with the pedals.

To stop and stand still, pedal slowly until the machine is almost ready to stop; then "catch the pedals half way," that is, stand on them, rising from the saddle, having the pedals at equal heights, and alternate the pressure. Hold the saddle firmly, pressing against both sides to feel the balance and to hold the balance by means of the saddle between the pedals with the weight on the feet.

As you catch the pedals, give the front wheel a sudden twist towards the back pedal, which will prevent the bicycle from falling on that side; then control the balance by the weight on the other pedal, and if necessary restore balance by a quick twist of the front wheel. The best way to practise this is to stop near a smooth wall, and use that to assist to steady the balance.

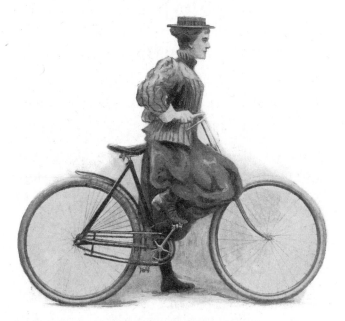

CORRECT MOUNTING POSITION.

Two people can stop and stand still in this way, crossing hands as in skating, gripping the inner handles of the bicycles, and stopping by holding the pedals and controlling the front wheels by the handles, using the outer hand. This makes a very pretty and effective pause.

Numbness undoubtedly comes from interrupted circulation, caused either by the clothing or the method of working. Numbness of the hands and fingers may be traced generally to tight clothing, and after all surface pressure is removed may safely be attributed to a too tight gripping of the handles. A large soft glove often aids to prevent numbness of the fingers; if gloves are not worn, the hand is apt to grasp too closely. Change of position, too, will tend to counteract numbness. It is not well to work too long at a time without a rest, if there is any tendency of this kind. Walk up hill or on the level to restore the circulation.

Numbness of the foot can be caused by surface pressure, the shoes, or the saddle. Sitting too close to the saddle while working, instead of carrying the weight on the pedals, is apt to produce numbness of the feet. Garters or belts will have the same effect, and must be watched and regulated. A shoe adapted for walking is not at all suitable for serious bicycle exercise; the strains and pressure all come in the wrong places, and confine and numb the feet. Free ankle movement is imperative, and freedom for the lower muscles of the calf of the leg; room for the feet, and especially for the toes to spread and to assist in pressing the pedal. The sole of the shoe should be stiff, to prevent bruises from the pedals or from irregularities on the ground.

Concussion and a consequent vibratory movement of the bicycle are impossible to avoid, but they need not affect the wheeler injuriously. Numbness is sometimes due to a condition of the nerves of the parts affected by the vibratory movement. To prevent this condition of affairs, never wheel with the weight on the hands, nor grip the handles of the handle-bars too tight. Rest the hands lightly on the handles, and be prepared to squeeze hard when necessary. Study the best position and most convenient height for the hands when the machine is best under control, and the jar and vibration are not perceived. All joints of wrist, elbow, and shoulder should transmit any motion, not locate it, by being fixed or rigid at any point.

The tire of the wheel should not be hard, nor should the saddle be fitted with springs; and it should be so placed as to allow the rider to rise easily on the pedals for rough wheeling. These rules being observed, serious danger from this cause need not be apprehended.

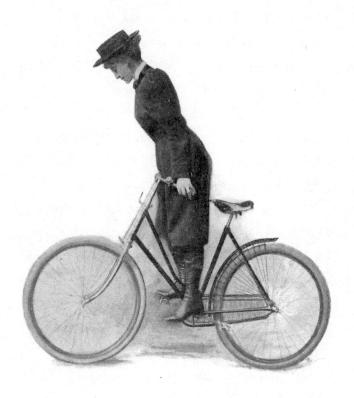

Mounting—second position.

Wheeling over cobble-stone pavement or over good Belgian blocks produces a marked vibration in the bicycle. It would be a satisfactory test for adjustment of position to be able to wheel over such a surface with comfort, feeling the vibration of the bicycle hardly at all.

The difficulty experienced in wheeling over rough surface is caused by lack of confidence and by general stiffness of all the muscles, which causes the full force of the vibration to be felt. In carrying the weight on the pedals, the vibration is less intensely felt. To grip the handles for rough surface riding is almost involuntary, but it is accompanied by acute discomfort from vibration. Pedal work only will meet this difficulty.

There are different methods of mounting. The pedal mount is usually the one first attempted on a drop-frame bicycle; the mount over the wheel on a diamond-frame.

The diamond-frame mount from the peg is made in this way: Standing directly behind the machine, the handles of the handle-bars are grasped firmly. One foot is placed on the peg, and the wheel inclined away from that foot; the foot on the ground gives a shove, and the bicycle moves off, carrying the weight on the peg; and the other foot swings forward to catch the pedal, which was a little behind the top of the circle on starting.

The drop-frame has several rather pretty pedal mounts and vaults. In one, the bars are held, and the machine is started. Watch the rhythm of the pedal, and as it passes the top of the stroke, incline the machine away from you, place the other foot on the pedal, swing the foot next the machine over in front, and catch the other pedal as it rises; then sit easily on the saddle. The vault is made after starting the machine, running or hurrying along, and springing from the ground to the saddle, using the handles to help. The pedals are found after being seated on the saddle; and the machine moves with the momentum given it in running before rising in the vault.

There is a mount from the pedal on the same side on which you are standing. Start the bicycle, and keep along with it, watching the pedals. As the pedal near you comes up and over the top of the curve, step on it with the outside foot, inclining the machine well away from you; at the same time the weight will carry the pedal around with you, and as it rises, the other pedal and the saddle can be found. The same mount may be made without starting the machine. Hold the machine inclined from you; place the outside foot against the pedal until it is at its furthest point away from you; hold the bicycle firmly, and step on, swinging the foot off the ground around to the other pedal, in front of the saddle, not behind it. On the diamond-frame, the same mount is made, only the foot is swung behind the saddle, not in front of it, as is possible on the drop-frame machine.

To stop the bicycle with another person on it, grasp the handle-bars, and take hold of the shoulder of the person propelling the bicycle, if necessary.

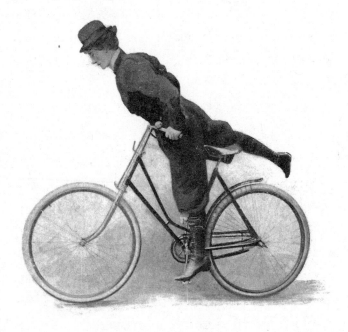

DISMOUNTING OVER THE WHEEL.

CHAPTER 11

DRESS

The matter of dress for bicycling is quite important from the hygienic standpoint.

Clothing should be most carefully selected, with the view to an equal distribution of weight and an even thickness of material; it should have no constricting, no tight bands anywhere, but should permit of absolute freedom of movement, and be warm enough to prevent chilling through too great radiation of heat, yet porous enough to allow of free evaporation.

All seasons of the year permit of cycling; the bicyclist therefore has opportunity for much variety in dress. The essentials are knickerbockers, shirtwaist, stockings, shoes, gaiters, sweater, coat, no skirt, or skirt with length decided by individual preference, hat and gloves.

The knickerbockers should be very carefully cut; smooth and tight just over the top of the hips, and fitting easily below; not full or gathered; full at the knees, and boxed or finished with a band and button and button-hole; nothing elastic on any account. The stockings should be worn folded on the boxed part of the knickerbockers, below the knees, and rolled down and held by the band of the knickerbockers, being fastened below. This arrangement does away with garters, which compress surface circulation, or pull if attached at the waist, causing pressure where they pull, and are most objectionable for many reasons. The knickerbockers should be made of cloth or woollen material.

The shirt-waist should have wristbands or sleeves finished to open a little way, and button; the neck finished with a band, with a detachable collar of the same material. The body of the waist should be shaped to the figure at the sides and back, gathered slightly in the front, and finished at the waist-line without a band, and may be of the same material as the rest of the suit. The knickerbockers should button to this waist, the places for the buttons being reinforced. The stockings should preferably be of wool, and of a seasonable weight.

The combination of knickerbockers, shirt-waist, and stockings forms the essential part of a cycling costume. A union under-garment may be worn and the knicker-bocker suit; over this a coat and a skirt if desired, with a sweater for an extra wrap.

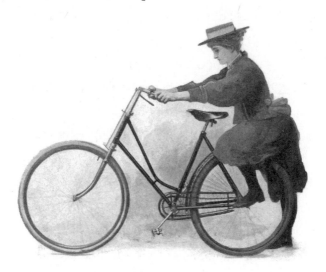

MOUNTING OVER THE WHEEL FROM PEG.

Bicycling is warm work, and the clothing should always be rather light in weight. For touring it must all be carried on the wheel, and yet be heavy enough for comfort when not exercising, and not too heavy for work, and should, moreover, allow of adjustment for changes in temperature or for any required change in distribution. To this end, all the clothing should be of one color or of colors that look well together. The knickerbockers, waist, and skirt should match; then if the coat is removed, the costume looks complete. An outfit might consist of two suits complete, of different weights; sweaters of different weights; wool stockings, heavy and light, that will roll below the knee without being either bulky or tight.

The knickerbockers are better fastened with a button, the button being in just the right place, than with a strap and buckle, which is liable to be pulled too tight at times.

The shoes should be low, made of thin leather, laced well down toward the toe, with light uppers, and soles stiff yet flexible, and made with grooves to take the pedals and prevent slipping. Blocks or cleats on the soles to fit the pedals are sometimes preferred, but are hardly so good for general work.

The gaiters may be made of almost any suitable material, leather, canvas, or woollen, to match or contrast with the rest of the costume. They should fit easily around the ankle and over the instep, and should never, on any account, extend more than half way to the knee. The muscles of the calf of the leg must have room to work; and gaiters badly cut, or too tight or too long, would impede circulation and restrict muscular action.

The sweater should come well up around the neck, and pull down easily below the saddle; it is better too long than not long enough to cover the large muscular masses that have been at work, and may be turned up if in the way. It should slip on easily, and be soft and woolly, and not so cumbersome that the coat cannot slip on over it and be buttoned up to the throat.

The coat should be cut long-waisted, and easy across the shoulders, single-breasted, and made to button close to the throat; the collar to roll and remain open, but so cut that it may be easily turned up to the ears. The sleeves should be finished with two buttons and button-holes, so that they may be turned up a little if desired.

There are occasions when a covert coat made of close cloth may be useful, when out in very cold weather or standing in the wind without shelter; but it cannot be generally recommended.

Pockets in any part of the dress should be made of woollen material. Cotton retains moisture, and a cotton pocket or a pocket lined with cotton may become damp and clammy and cold, acting almost like a damp compress. The fewer pockets, the better; but a number are often found convenient. Everything if possible should be carried on the wheel, not in the pockets. Metal condenses moisture and interrupts evaporation.

As the skirt should always open at the side, and fasten with several buttons, a convenient pocket may be placed in the placket-hole; a watch-pocket in the skirt is a good thing, but the watch is better carried on the wheel; and a pocket should be set aside for matches, where they may always be found quickly.

Collars and cuffs of linen or of celluloid, of silk or of the same material as the suit, may be used for touring; but soft neckwear should be worn if possible.

If a neck-muffler is worn, it should be of cashmere, not of silk.

Neatness is most important. Each article of dress should be carefully adjusted and fastened. Never use pins or put things carelessly together, hoping they will stay, but be sure that every article of dress fits and is securely fastened, and it will never need a thought after it is in place.

In warm weather gloves with one button are most comfortable; for cooler weather, four buttons, fastened about the wrists, keep the hands warm.

The adjustment of the covering of wrists and ankles makes the greatest difference in comfort in wheeling. In cold weather, hands and feet should be kept warm; in hot weather, it is comfortable to work with the cuffs turned back and wearing low shoes without gaiters. Indeed, in hot weather it is important not to encase the ankles in heavy boots or leggings, as these would ensure overheating.

The outfit may be completed with a number of hats—a light straw for summer, a soft felt for touring, and a small and becoming hat for the park. The hat should be chosen to stay on easily, and not pinned, but fastened under the hair with elastic, and the hair dressed to stand any amount of blowing about.

The skirt should not reach more than half way below the knee, and the hem and all seams should be finished on the outside; then there will be nothing to catch or pull. The width around the bottom may be a matter of choice, but the skirt need not fall behind the pedal when furthest back, and should be cut full enough in the front to permit the knees to work easily. The top of the skirt should take the place of a waistband, following the curves of the figure, made to flare at the top of the waist, and fitted snugly over the hips and hanging from them. It may be worn with or without a belt.

The coat should be long enough to touch the saddle or hang an inch or two below it, to protect all the vital organs and as much of the working masses of muscle as possible.

The sweater may be worn for coolness or warmth. As an outside garment, it allows the air to pass through its mesh easily; worn under another garment, it is very warm, retaining the heat.

The color of a bicycle suit may be chosen for the kind of work to be done; its texture may be decided suitable if, a piece being held over the mouth, it is possible to inhale and exhale through it easily. The cloth should be firm enough to stand wear and rough usage; smooth enough to shed dust easily; and of a quality that will stand being wet without shrinking, and will turn the rain if caught in a shower. It should be firm, elastic, soft; have what is known as substance; be very light in weight and yet not clinging; and possessing all these qualities, the ideal cloth for bicycling should not be so expensive that it cannot be renewed easily.

Simplicity in detail for any garment made to work in is always commendable, and a bicycle dress must be simple to be suitable.

A corset, if one is worn, should not extend below the waist-line, and should have elastic side-lacing.

To choose what to wear when the weather is changeable is rather difficult; and the bicyclist starting early in the morning for an all-day outing must expect changes of temperature during the day. Starting, the coat may be folded on the handles, and the sweater worn; later, as the sun grows warmer, the sweater may be removed; at the noonday halt, the coat may be donned while lunching, as it usually seems chilly coming under cover; later in the afternoon the sweater is again of use; and before the evening is advanced, the coat worn over the sweater often proves acceptable.

For touring, only an extra change of underwear, with a change of neckwear, is needed to carry on the wheel.

To look well at all times when bicycling, it is necessary to remember the possible conditions that may be encountered, and to wear no garment that may prove incongruous.

When touring, of course, fresh toilettes may be indulged in at the expense of extra luggage. The chief pleasure of bicycling is independence and the joy of being free; yet a long trip without access to the conveniences and even the luxuries of civilization, should not be attempted. A trunk may be sent home as soon as it has been proved unnecessary, or sent ahead and met at intervals; but its non-arrival should never be allowed to disconcert the traveller.

It is an accepted fact that bicycling cannot be properly enjoyed unless the clothing is suitable. Of course, one can take a drop-frame bicycle, mount, and wheel slowly for a short distance, barring inconveniences, in ordinary dress; so can one swim a little if unexpectedly placed in the water. Bicycling requires the same freedom of movement that swimming does, and the dress must not hamper or hinder.

CHAPTER 12

WATCH AND CYCLOMETER

Suitably attired, with a bicycle of the latest model and most perfect construction, it matters little whether the residence be in town or country, for the largest city is soon left behind. The country, when the highway ceases to be passable, is easily travers-able on the foot-trodden pathway beside it. Wherever the foot has trodden, the wheel may follow, if the path be well defined; and as the wheel can be carried easily, there is no limit but the limit of endurance in crossing country that cannot be wheeled over. But in order to cover distance without dismounting and within a time limit, where the speed attained is an element to be considered, good roads should be chosen.

The bicycle multiplies our power of advancing by five. One who can walk three miles in an hour can wheel fifteen miles on a bicycle, given all the conditions necessary to attain that speed for the period of an hour. The wonderful speed of the running and sprinting athlete is again multiplied by five, for a short time, in the contests where wheeling records are made.

While increasing the distance travelled the bicycle has greatly decreased the time limit. A person travelling afoot at the rate of three miles an hour (the average walking gait) covers a mile in twenty minutes, and at the end of an hour is not more than three miles from the starting point. On a bicycle a mile is covered usually in four minutes or less. The average distance, owing to the varied resistance met, is not usually so great; and more power may be expended in the hour than is required to walk three miles in the same length of time. Six miles may be the record for an hour on a wheel, and yet the amount of work done be very great. Until the position is adjusted to suit individual requirements, the output of power to accomplish a certain distance, even though it be a short one, is necessarily great. Considerable study is necessary to work out the perfect individual adjustment of the bicycle, weight of clothing, and amount of practice requisite to easy, rhythmical movement; but that once attained, the world lies before you.

Bicycling trains and quickens the perceptions; it cultivates and develops courage, judgment, and discrimination as well as prompt decision and quick and accurate sight. The hand follows the eye without effort; and the machine responds to each impression received without conscious expenditure of power.

To cyclists is due the keen public interest recently aroused in good roadways and in legislation to effect their construction, and the consequent improvement in public highways. For years the amateur cyclists of the country labored to this end in the interest of the sport, the League of American Wheelmen intelligently preparing the minds of the public on the subject.

To be accomplished as a bicyclist means something more than knowing how to wheel a bicycle and to be able to get about on it. It is necessary besides to keep informed of the laws and ordinances relating to bicycles and to vehicles in general; to possess a complete and accurate knowledge of the wheel as a machine; to be able to do for it all that can be done one's self or to direct another who has not this knowledge; to know the country travelled, know distance and direction; the use of map and compass, and how to travel without them, finding the direction by sun or stars, or even, if need be, without either; to understand the effect of time and season on the face of nature and to cultivate the senses of the woods.

If, while touring with a party, you find that you have missed the way in a strange country and that something about the bicycle has given out, calm decision is requisite. Estimate your resources, and keep quiet. Do not try to find your party; let them find you. Study your wheel-tracks; if off the line of travel, follow them carefully to where they join the tracks of your companions. Then wait until some one comes for you. Rest or be busy about your wheel. Do what you can easily, not to be tired and worn out when your companions find you. It is seldom wise to try and walk after the party; the only object in moving would be to keep warm, for a chill must be avoided.

There is a wonderful difference in the distances covered under different conditions. Winds, adverse or favorable, affect the bicyclist more than anything else. An unfavorable wind is one directly ahead or that can be felt on either cheek while advancing. A favorable wind is one that blows on the back, or cannot be felt on either cheek while looking ahead. A wind blowing directly at right angles with the direction of the wheel is a favorable wind; you unconsciously balance against it, and the bicycle glides forward under pressure as a boat does with the sail trimmed in.

When starting out, note the weather conditions; what the prevailing winds are and what the changes are likely to be during the time you expect to be on your bicycle. If the wind is west or northwest, do not take that direction for the run out, unless the trip is to be a short one. Always try to have the wind with you, both going and returning. Learn the peculiarities of the weather and study the government weather reports; they are of quite as much assistance to the bicyclist as to the mariner who knows how to use them; for winds frequently change their direction, and the indications for such changes should be sought and studied.

If a short trip is planned, as the wind is not likely to change during the run, start out against the wind; that is, plan to do the hardest work first, and let the wind help on the return. Avoid hard work whenever possible.

Hill-climbing against the wind is the hardest kind of work; with the wind to assist, even quite steep hills may often be coasted part of the way up, and all easy grades taken with the feet off the pedals. Coasting should be indulged in with discretion, or the bicycle may run away with you. Check speed at the first indication that the wheel is escaping control by applying the brake and catching the pedal, back pedaling at the same time. On a public road, the bicycle should never be beyond control.

To thoroughly enjoy an outing, road, direction, and atmospheric conditions should be studied. If you are out for several hours' spin in chilly weather, there is little pleasure to be had in exploring; but in weather when the temperature permits of stops without danger to health, frequent dismounts and short-distance trips across country are enjoyable. One of the pleasures of bicyclists is the good fellowship existing between them, which is rarely disturbed. On the bicycle conversation is interrupted by long pauses, by intervals of silence, when each rider is alone, with opportunity for reflection and mental expansion.

On long trips note first the general direction of the road, the wind, and the sun; try to have the wind with you and the sun behind you for the better part of the day. Be able to change your plans quickly to meet changed conditions, and have a reserve of grit to fall back on if things do not go quite to your liking. Dressed for bicycling, it matters little whether it rains or shines; but wind, sand, and stones make impossible conditions for the bicyclist. When wind has reached a certain velocity, wheeling becomes unsafe. Mud causes the wheels to slip and prevents them from turning; sand does the same. A surface offering little or no resistance is impossible. Stones are dangerously liable to cause spills, while ruts and bumps twist the bicycle and are apt to throw the rider.

In the autumn months, when the sun sets early, a lantern should be provided even when it seems an absurdly unnecessary encumbrance; for a town or village where the ordinances are strict may lie on the route, and the unlucky bicyclist without a light must go afoot.

Of course, speeding cannot be attempted with the bicycle encumbered; but with all the extras, a good average speed may be maintained. The bicyclist wishing for freedom from all encumbrance is apt to forget unpleasant possibilities. A punctured tire thirty miles from anything is such a possibility; so, though the tool-kit weighs something, it can never prudently be dispensed with.

Have the bicycle all ready, and start free from care and with a quiet mind, after a last careful and reassuring inspection of the machine. Starting from a town with a perfectly running machine, the attention is first directed to getting into the country easily, either by train or by wheeling. In wheeling, streets free from traffic and with the best possible surfaces should be chosen.

Country wheeling is often good when city work is impossible. The dangers of city wheeling are traffic, car tracks, and mud. City mud is usually of a greasy nature, very difficult to wheel over. Even pedaling is very necessary, and uneven pressure on the pedals means a side spill.

In wheeling over mud, never attempt to control the machine by the front wheel; it must be controlled by the pedals. If too much pressure is used, there is nothing left but to step off. Do not try to recover by means of the front wheel; the attempt will be useless, and a fall can be avoided only by stepping off. Keep the front wheel steady, and rely on the weight-carrying wheel to take you clear of the mud. Keep a sharp lookout, and travel slowly. Any one can make a bicycle go.

Get out of town, and then be ready to pedal up to

time on the first clear stretch of good road. Make time, but never hurry. Never work hard over hill-work or try to go fast against the wind. When using side-paths, always recollect they may be protected by local ordinances. Keep posted on the law of the road, taking to the highway on approaching towns and villages. If the work is hard, travel slowly, and look ahead. Two good rules are—To travel fast, look well ahead; and watch the ground when there is a hard bit of road to pass over.

A good stiff pull against the wind can be accomplished easily, really easily, if you take your time, giving full attention to pedaling, and keeping the eyes a short distance ahead of the wheel. It is much easier to rest on the bicycle by slowing than to dismount. In cold weather, never stop without seeking shelter, at least the lee of bank or wall; and keep away from a fire, as it renders one liable to take cold. Nothing is so dangerous in frosty weather as a pause of even a few minutes dismounted.

In warm weather, it is permissible to drink water when wheeling; but it should be remembered that the bicyclist passes through all sorts of country, and the water may sometimes be anything but drinkable from a sanitary point of view, even causing typhoid and other fevers. Water that has been boiled is unpalatable, but it is safe; boiled and cooled, it may be rendered more palatable by shaking it or pouring it from one pitcher to another to mix air with it. Ice in water is another source of danger. The water, after being boiled or filtered, should be placed in bottles with absorbent cotton for stoppers, and cooled by being placed on ice. Muddy water may be cleansed with a piece of alum. If a lump of alum is stirred about for a second or two in a pail or pitcher of muddy water, and then the water allowed to settle, it will be found fit to boil for drinking. Bottled waters are safest when the country is unknown or when there is doubt as to the purity of the local supply; but failing these, the precautions mentioned will ensure safety.

Never prolong bicycle exercise without eating, and never work after a hearty meal; but the consumption of a couple of sandwiches at noon cannot be regarded as a serious meal; and it is often better to push on after a short halt, moving slowly, than to sit around on rocks or stumps to wait for a proper digestive period to elapse. It is well to have a small reserve supply of food, such as chocolate or beef tablets, to tide one over a prolonged period between meals. Milk and bread and cheese are good to take as an extra meal. Never work hungry if it can be avoided; the bicycle will lag, and the cyclist wonder at being weary. Keep up the food supply by all means, for fatigue sets in quickly with the desire for food, and the system quickly becomes enfeebled.

The cyclometer registers each revolution of the wheel, and by an ingenious mechanism the dial gives the record in miles. There is a great temptation to roll up miles, that the cyclometer may make a good showing; indeed, this striving after mileage often becomes a ruling passion, interfering with the real pleasures of the sport.

The pedestrian, accustomed to noting distances, can usually judge the rate or pace travelled, and decide very accurately upon the distance traversed, with only the time as a guide; for the pace, so many miles an hour, multiplied by the number of hours, gives the distance.

On the bicycle the pace is very easily estimated in a similar manner. Count the strokes per minute as each knee rises, divide that by two, and you have the number of revolutions of the crank. The gear gives the diameter of the wheel larger than the one on the bicycle; sixty-four gear, for instance, means that the crank revolution covers a distance equal to a wheel with a diameter of sixty-four inches. The circumference of a wheel is three times its diameter; and 64 multiplied by 3 equals 192 inches measured on the ground for one revolution of the crank. Multiply the distance measured on the ground by the crank revolution by the number of strokes made per minute, divide by twelve to give the number of feet the crank has covered in one revolution, and you have the distance in feet travelled per minute. To find the rate of miles per hour, multiply that result by 60 to find the number of feet travelled per hour, and divide the result by 5280, the number of feet in a mile. The watch should have a second hand for bicycle work. The cyclometer taken for five minutes, then multiplied by twelve, gives the rate of mileage per hour, a very convenient way of ascertaining the rate of speed per hour.

It is well to know the rhythm of stroke of a certain rate per hour, for it is often of assistance in determining distance, and will frequently prevent a hurry when train connections are to be made, by assuring you that you are easily travelling a pace that will take you to your destination on time.

The alertness and quickness of perception that bicycling cultivates seem marvellous. A road, previously accepted as ordinarily good, becomes full of pitfalls that the wary learn to avoid. Slippery or uneven surfaces, tacks and broken glass, are to be noted and avoided, inequalities allowed for, and preparation made to overcome the tendency of the machine on unexpected hard bits of road.

One of the dangers of sidepath wheeling often encountered is a slippery spot or a place where the surface may give way, such as the edge of a bank along which the path runs, with a fence on the other side. Here, if the bicycle slips, the bicyclist is pretty sure to be thrown against the fence. In sidepath wheeling a sharp lookout must be kept for these slippery spots and weak edges, and also for stones or stumps that run through the uneven surface.

A first coast on a hill whose pitch has been miscalculated, and which proves steeper than was anticipated, is a terrible surprise. To find one's self clinging desperately to a runaway machine, with no hope save in the ascending grade that seems so far away, is anything but a pleasant experience. In such case sit still, hold fast, keep straight, and if nothing is in the way to collide with, there is hope, barring unexpected surface obstacles. The coaster's safety in steering lies in swaying; the pedals are out of the question, and the front wheel is better undisturbed. A slight inclination to either side will alter the course of the bicycle without interfering with balance or momentum, and the hands can be ready, gripping hard, to keep the wheel steady.

In coasting, sit well in the saddle, letting that take the whole weight, and do not push too hard with the feet on the coasters. The feet should not be braced against the coasters, but should rest easily against them with an even pressure.

To learn to coast, practise at first either on a slight or a small grade; another way is to get up speed on the level, and take one foot off at the time. The most marvellous experience of bicycling is to have a wind carry you coasting up hill—a wind, too, that is seemingly adverse, or at least not directly favorable.

Trust to the map, the watch, and the cyclometer to locate your whereabouts, and do not place too much faith in answers to inquiries, unless you are speaking to a bicyclist; for people unaccustomed to accurate judgment differ greatly in their estimation of a given distance or a general direction. You need only stop three or four times in a mile or two, and inquire the way to a town say five or six miles distant, to be convinced of this fact.

CHAPTER 13

WOMEN AND TOOLS

Most women can sew on a button or run up a seam; sewing, in fact, is regarded rather as a feminine instinct than an art. There are many capable people in the world, both men and women, who can comprehend at a glance the use or the application of an article or an idea—people who instinctively use their eyes and hands with ease and accuracy; there are others who learn more slowly to use their mechanical senses; and there are also those whose attention has never been called to certain simple mechanical facts and details that they are quite capable of understanding. To all the mastery of these facts means an expenditure of more or less time, and in this busy world of ours, there is nothing so much appreciated or so carelessly wasted. It is my intention to place before my readers a few simple mechanical explanations.

I hold that any woman who is able to use a needle or scissors can use other tools equally well. It is a very important matter for a bicyclist to be acquainted with all parts of the bicycle, their uses and adjustment. Many a weary hour would be spared were a little proper attention given at the right time to your machine.

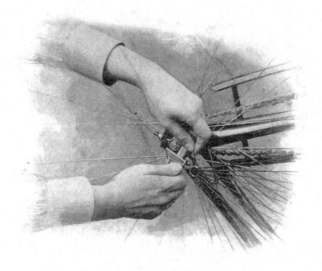

STARTING A NUT.

Ask any carriage maker or coachman, and he will tell you that everything on wheels needs attention. Any owner or lover of horses will say that horses require constant care. The bicyclist is the motor, the horse; the bicycle, the vehicle. These ideas should remain distinct. When you mount a wheel, you do not mount an iron horse; you are a human propelling power, and the bicycle is a carriage.

It is all important to work without unnecessary effort, and for this you must have a knowledge of bicycle construction, how to make the machine run smoothly, and how not to injure the human motor or the mechanism. The human body is so beautifully self-adjustable that it may be safely attributed to ignorance or neglect if anything goes wrong with it. Attention should always be paid at the right time to nature's warnings; they are danger-signals, and if disregarded, unpleasant results are sure to follow. A little common-sense goes far; and with that and a right knowledge—not necessarily an extensive knowledge—of the working of the human machine, there need be little to fear from injuries resulting from athletic exercise.

The amount of work different individuals can perform, of course, varies. Find out how much work you ought to do, and do it. A physician is the only competent judge of your limitations. Never attempt any new form of exercise without being examined for it. Sensible people when they purchase a horse require a veterinary certificate to accompany the guarantee; and the work the horse is to do is planned according to the ascertained amount the animal is capable of performing. If it is right for you to wheel but five miles every other day, and at a certain hour only, it does not follow that that is always to be your limit. Practice accomplishes great results; and the strength and endurance that come of exercise taken regularly, under proper conditions, seems marvellous to those who, after a course of proper preparation, attempt and accomplish with pleasure and ease what at first seemed impossible. It is hard, of course, to see some one else do what you would like to do and cannot; but it is weak not to be able to say, "I have done enough, and I must stop." There are many other people similarly placed.

The bicycle may be so adapted and adjusted as to enable bicyclists of different powers to work together and enjoy a fair amount of sociability; for if one has wheeled around the world, why should that spoil one's pleasure in wheeling around a block? To wheel alone is not much pleasure. Find some one to wheel around the and combinations of movements must be learned; they cannot be acquired hurriedly with good results. People who can work well are usually patient with a beginner who is doing his best, knowing themselves what it means to work hard and to face disappointment and failure and what is involved in repeated effort. The ambitious are liable to over-exertion, the timid not to practice enough.

There is much prejudice against athletic exercise for women and girls, many believing that nothing of the kind can be done without over-doing; but there is a right way of going about athletics as everything else. Prejudice can be removed only by showing good results, and good results can be accomplished only by work done under proper restrictions. To do a thing easily is to do it gracefully; and grace, without properly balanced muscular action, is impossible; grace is the embodiment of balance, strength, and intelligence. Jerky movement indicates lack of muscular development and training.

The human machine is capable of a seemingly unlimited series of muscular movements and combined muscular motions. Any training or practice of mind or muscles assists to fit them for new combinations. But little time is necessary to learn to know how to do and what to do, though the subjects to be considered, mechanics and physiology, are exhaustive and extensive in their range.

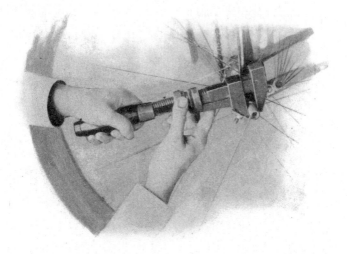

ADJUSTING A WRENCH.

It is always a pleasure to do a thing well, whether it is handling a needle or using a screw-driver; and the art of using either successfully is not difficult to acquire. With the bicycle it is necessary to know what to do; the human motor, unless pushed beyond reasonable limits, is self-adjusting. Over-taxing is the result often of too great ambition, of failure to keep in view the proper aim of exercise, and sacrificing health and ultimate success for passing vanity. The bicycle is but the means to the end, first of all, of health—health of mind and body. The human mechanism is far more difficult to adjust when out of order than the mechanism of the bicycle. In bicycling, the two machines are one and interdependent. The foot on the pedal pushing the crank is but one point of application of power conveyed by a series of levers, actuated by muscles, controlled by nerves, supplied and directed by accumulated power.

We hear of horse-power as a unit; we have also human power—the amount of power the average individual can exercise. Food supplies material to be converted into power, stored and transmuted in the human system either for use or waste, as the case may be. Energy or power, unless applied within a specified time, is given off as heat, etc. Less food is needed, loss of appetite follows, if too little work is done. The muscular tissues become almost useless, it is an effort to do any kind of work; the power is not there. By gradual and persistent practice, strength is acquired, and power stored in reserve. Exercise tends to strengthen, not to weaken; over-exercise uses up stored power and newly acquired power as well; longer periods of rest are needed to renew the wasted tissues than is necessary when exercise is not carried to excess. It must be kept in mind when bicycling that rider and wheel are a complete, compound, combined mechanism, and mechanically inseparable. The wheeler's weight, when shifted or inclined, affects his equilibrium, and wheeler and bicycle are as much one as a skater and his skates.

Levers and their application; power, stored, distributed, or wasted; how to prevent waste and acquire reserve; proper adjustment to mechanical environment, translated to mean the use of a few common tools, and their application to the adjustment of the bicycle; and the care, adjustment, and proper preparation of the machine for work, are points of such importance that too much stress cannot be laid on them. A little thought, a little attention at the right time, prepares for emergencies, for cheerful work, and for the enjoyment of the exercise, and the health and accumulated benefits sure to follow.

CHAPTER 14

TOOLS AND HOW TO USE THEM

"A nut is a piece of metal adapted to screw on the end of a bolt." "A bolt is a stout metallic pin adapted for holding objects together." The nut is to the bolt what the knot is to the thread, to keep it from slipping through. Iron and steel are fibrous materials, and very hard; though strong, they are also brittle. Indeed, these metals, and metals generally, resemble molasses candy in their nature more than any other familiar substance that will serve for illustration. When heated, they become soft and liquid; when cold, they are tough, hard, and even brittle. A few powerful, sharp blows with a heavy object are enough to fracture a piece of metal. Direct, heavy blows or tapping on the end of a bolt will flatten and alter its shape sufficiently to cause the edges to project, a very little seemingly, but enough to render it useless.

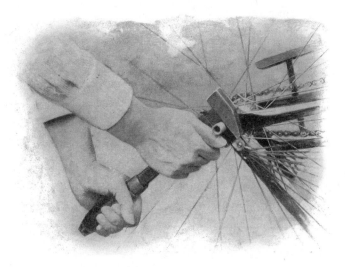

Applying power.

If you wish to remove a bolt that seems to fit too tight and resists ordinary methods, place the nut on the bolt, and screw it on level, so that the end of the bolt will be flush or even with the top of the nut. Then lay your piece of wood, quite smooth and flat, on the nut and bolt, covering both, and hammer gently on that with a heavy hammer, with gentle, short, sharp, even strokes. The most obstinate bolt will usually yield to this method of persuasion. Should a burr have formed on the end of a bolt, a file is necessary to remove it; and filing off a burr is a somewhat lengthy and tedious operation.

Unscrew a nut gently and examine it. On the inside will be found a spiral groove and a spiral ridge or thread. Examine the bolt, and observe a similar spiral groove and thread. These, when screwed together, prevent slipping, and the nut cannot be pulled or pushed off. To remove the nut, it is necessary to turn it; and always turn one way, from left to right, if the nut lies uppermost.

To keep a nut from unscrewing by jarring, etc., screw it down until it jams, as it is called, firmly against the surface it rests on. If screwed too tight, it will burst or break the thread, or if enough force is applied the bolt may break. This hardly seems possible until we realize that in the wrench we possess a very powerful lever, capable of destroying quite a large bolt and its accompanying nut. If pains be taken always to start a nut on square and to turn gently and firmly and not too fast, the previous instructions may prove unnecessary.

There are usually two kinds of wrench in a bicycle outfit—an adjustable wrench with sliding jaw, and one or more key-wrenches, so called because made to fit particular parts of the machine, and to be used for them only. The adjustable wrench with sliding jaw should be used with the pressure or pull coming on the angle of the head, and the sliding jaw so placed as to hold its position, the wrench applied so that the greatest strain is taken at the strongest part; then the faces of the jaw keep smooth and true, and will not deface the plating or polish of the machine.

There is another point to note—that a properly adjusted wrench starts a nut easily, while if the strain is taken on the movable jaw of the wrench, there is give enough in the wrench itself to prevent the nut from starting, and the wrench slips off the nut without effecting its object. The handle of the wrench acts as a lever, and the head of the wrench forms a right angle with the handle; it is here that the power is centred, not at the angle made by the movable jaw. Of course, this position seems the reverse of proper until it is analyzed; but once understood and adopted, it will prove most effective.

There are various screws in and about the machine. A screw is defined as a bolt or bar having a thread cut upon it spirally, so that it will enter a hole in which a corresponding spiral groove and thread have been cut, or on which they will be formed by the screw entering the hole. The thread and screw interwind and prevent the screw from being withdrawn unless it is turned. To turn the screw, a notch is cut on one end, which is made flat for that purpose, and the other end of the screw is pointed, to enable it to enter the hole easily. After a screw is placed and started in its proper hole, it is only necessary to turn it until it is driven home. To turn the screw, a short bar is flattened thin to enter the notch on the end of the screw.

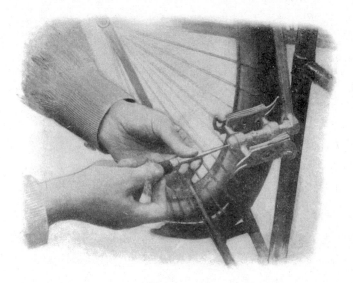

SCREWING UP.

The screw-driver should be held and turned with one hand, and steadied and guided with the other. Metal is not so hard but that the leverage of the screw-driver is enough to bend the notches on the end of a screw, and thus render it useless. The question may be raised, why are not screws made harder? If metal is tempered too hard, it becomes brittle, and flies. A well-tempered screw should be neither too hard nor too soft, but adapted for its particular use or position.

A screw should always be made clean before it is screwed home, any particle of dust or rust being liable to injure the thread and spoil the screw. If the screw is oily or greasy, it will work loose. All screws, bolts, etc., therefore, should be carefully wiped, and never placed where there is any chance for even a little dust to settle upon them. A nut with a small grain of sand inside will burst or break the thread of the bolt.

Bolts and screws are used to hold different parts together or in place and to give strength and firmness.

There is usually an oil-can belonging to every machine, and a bicycle should be provided with a good one, small, light, and easily carried; and special care should be taken that it does not leak. A greasy oilcan is unpleasant to handle and almost useless, as it cannot be handled properly. The least possible amount of oil that can be used is the proper quantity. Greasy bearings only collect dust, and the dust follows the oil back into the friction surfaces, where its presence is always undesirable.

Two kinds of lubricant are used on a bicycle—oil and graphite. A lubricant is used to diminish friction where two or more surfaces move over each other. If these surfaces are of the same material and the same degree of hardness, they do not slip; but the unevennesses of the surfaces engage each other and cause resistance, which produces friction, and friction causes heat, and the parts move more and more slowly, until at last they stop. Now, if a substance of a different character, like oil or graphite, is introduced between the moving surfaces, it forms little cushions, which prevent the two surfaces from coming into close contact; and, as the oil or graphite splits up readily into minute particles, the surfaces slip upon that, instead of holding fast. A smooth surface of metal is full of inequalities, perceptible when magnified, and slipping past each other with as much difficulty as would surfaces of sand paper. Only oil of the best quality and pure graphite should be used. Nothing sticky or gritty in its nature should be allowed near bearing surfaces.

The pump is an all-important and indispensable adjunct of the pneumatic tire. Each tire is fitted with a valve, and accompanied by a pump with which to inflate it. A valve is a lifting, sliding cover, connected with an aperture to prevent the passage of air or other fluids, and so constructed that the pump forces the cover down, and the air pushes past. The cover is held in place by a spring and air pressure, and, fitting tightly against a washer of some soft, impervious material, makes an air-tight joint, and will not move unless displaced. The pump itself is fitted with a valve to fill its cylinder or barrel with air, and to hold the air after the cylinder is full and when the plunger of the pump is forcing the air out of it again. A flexible tube coupling is used to connect the pump-barrel with the valve of the tire.

The valves are of many patterns and sizes, and there are pumps made to fit special tires, and pumps that will in a manner suit almost any ordinary valve. It is most important to note that all the washers about the pump and valves are in place. Deflated tires are often caused by a misplaced washer; and though valves are so constructed that it is not easy to disturb the washers, still it is well to know where they are and when they require attention. Washers wear out and require renewing, and sometimes a defective washer should be replaced; they are usually made of rubber or leather, but metal washers are sometimes used where there is much pressure or friction.

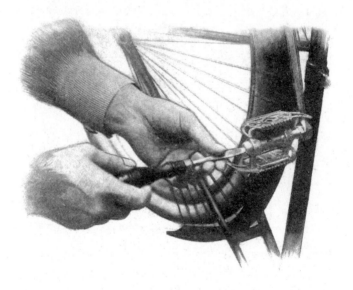

UNSCREWING.

The metal used in bicycle construction must be finished, smoothed, and prepared to resist the corroding effects of the atmosphere and to present an attractive and durable exterior. The metal used for the different parts must be smoothed and polished; all foreign substances, like grease, removed from their surface by a chemical process; and lastly a coating of nickel deposited on the surface by means of electricity. The nickel in this way becomes a part of the original metal, and protects its surface from rust and corrosion. A well-nickeled piece of metal, beautifully polished, and kept free from finger marks, loses its lustre only when neglected. Of course, there are other ways of finishing the surface of the metal parts of the bicycle; other plating metal may be substituted for the nickel, and other finish than polish used.

Light wheels cannot be recommended for rough country or for very fast work over only moderately good roads. A certain weight of material has been taken from the bicycle to make it light; the machine begins to lose its rigidity and consequently its accuracy, and cannot maintain its direction, but wavers, and really travels further to attain a given distance. The weight of a bicycle should depend on the roads it is to cover and the purposes it is to serve. Very light wheels wear out quickly; they cannot stand the strain of practice. Beginners, therefore, should choose a wheel that can endure the handling they will give it.

A very light, well-made, and delicately adjusted bicycle can carry a skilled cyclist anywhere; but a light wheel sooner loses its accuracy, and is then more difficult to work than a heavier wheel that runs true. Heavy wheels are not to be endured; light wheels, too light wheels, not to be encouraged.

CHAPTER 15

SOLVING A PROBLEM

When choosing a wheel, you should know what you want and why you want it. Machines are built for special purposes, and any reliable dealer can help you in selecting a machine and will guarantee satisfaction. Bicycles wear out, of course, but with proper care they may be made to last a long time.

Careful examination of your wheel should always be made before starting for even a short ride; and on returning it is well to test gear and pedals, to look at spokes and tires. Any needed repair can be noted, and attended to at convenience. Always examine your bicycle thoroughly after a collision, for shocks are dangerous even to the toughest metal, and such precaution may prevent a serious accident.

On returning from a ride the wheel should have a thorough going over, the enamel dusted, and any mud washed off with a wet sponge. The chain, if your machine has one, should be taken off every two or three hundred miles of dusty road, and soaked in kerosene over night; the nickel or metal well dusted, rubbed with a chamois, and polished; and all the bearings, axles, and gear carefully wiped, and dust and grit removed. Then the chain should be replaced, oiled, graphited, and the bearings oiled.

The chain is a complicated mechanism, consisting of many repetitions of parts; it should be kept clean and well lubricated. To apply graphite, turn the wheel upside down, hold the graphite still against the chain, and turn the wheel. The oil is needed in the joints of the chain; the graphite where the chain engages the cogs. The other parts used for applying power need the usual care given to the best machines—absolute cleanliness, freedom from grit, and thorough lubrication.

The chain is at present a mechanical detail only, and the application of power to the wheel capable of a great variety of forms. The principle remains the same, the application of power; the mechanical contrivance for transmitting it is a detail of construction. The difference of individuality can be compensated for in the length of the lever, size and number of gear, size of wheel, diameter of wheel, and width of tread.

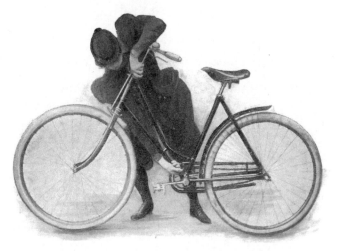

PREPARING TO TURN THE BICYCLE OVER.

The ideal machine requires little adjustment. The less the screws, the nuts, and the bearings are wrenched, the more perfect is the machine, the more free from wear and dents and scratches. To apply a wrench is a serious responsibility that should not be undertaken lightly. It seems easy, and yet skilled men are employed just for that kind of work, for it is work requiring the precision of the trained mechanic.

After purchasing a watch, the owner does not at once investigate the machinery; yet many, because the tools are at hand, are tempted to experiment on a bicycle. A bicycle, like a watch, should be ready to run, and only require winding up to keep it going. It should be adjusted; and if it needs regulating, this should be done by people who understand the machine and have the requisite knowledge and responsibility to do well what is to be done. Two rules may be laid down for one who does not study mechanical details—never to touch the bicycle except to ride it; and never to let any one else touch it who has not skill and experience.

This practice will prove satisfactory until some day, miles from home, the bicycle will not go; you carry it more miles to the nearest conveyance, and send it home. There you have it examined, and find that a touch sets it free; just as sometimes, when your watch will not go, you take it to a watchmaker, and he examines it, winds it up, and hands it back, telling you there is no charge. After learning to wheel a bicycle, therefore, the next step should be to learn to care for it. Unless somewhat familiar with machinery, it is bewildering to contemplate taking the thing apart and putting all those parts together again; even more bewildering is it, having taken the thing apart, not to be able to put it together. In such case, there is nothing to do but to gather the pieces of the puzzle, and send them to be set up. If in this extremity a friend who knows all about a bicycle should offer assistance, it is well to hear what he has to say before he undertakes the work. "I do not think your wheel is just like mine," perhaps, or "Where do these things belong?" is enough for the wise. Better send to the shop for a machinist at once. All the parts of the bicycle are made to go together in one way, and any attempt at experiment may injure the mechanism.

When you undertake to investigate a bicycle for the first time, take an old one as a subject, and endeavor to put it in perfect running order. If an old bicycle cannot be had, proceed with much circumspection. Go where you will be undisturbed, where there is plenty of room, and where a key may be turned if there is possibility of interruption. There is sure to be some oil and grease spattered about, in spite of the utmost care, and it is well to remember this while making preparations. Have ready a pile of old newspapers, some cups, plates, and boxes, and a painting apron if you possess one; if not an old skirt and apron, and sleeves well rolled up. For tools, a monkey-wrench, two or three screw-drivers, large as well as small, a hammer, one or two pieces of wood, the bicycle kit, oil, graphite, a can of kerosene, some cheesecloth and canton flannel, and a large wooden box.

Take two newspapers folded in half, and put them on the floor for the saddle and handle-bars; then turn the bicycle upside down, and arrange the newspapers under the saddle and handles. If there is a bell, take it off, or place a block under the opposite end of the bar to balance it. Before turning the bicycle over, remove the lantern, if there is one on the bicycle, as the oil will be spilled out if the lamp is turned upside down.

Begin by carefully removing all mud and grit from the bicycle. Wear old gloves, and remove mud with the hand when possible, finishing with a cheesecloth duster and an old oily cloth. Go over all the joints where the wheels turn, and remove every particle of grit, then remove mud and dust.

An experienced worker, to save labor, cleans each piece as it comes off, but the beginner must work more slowly. Have ready a shallow box or tray to receive the parts as they are removed. Lay each part, as it is taken off, in the tray, with the oily side up, for a guide. First, remove the chain, turn it until the nut of the little screw-bolt is found. This little bolt forms one of the link-pins, and can be found quite readily. One end of the bolt has a screw-head notch, and the other a nut and thread. Use the small bicycle screw-wrench for this, a large screw-driver, and a small screw-driver to fit the screw. Turn the chain until the bolt is in a convenient position, then take the large screw-driver or a rod, and place through the spokes of the rear wheel, letting the bar rest on the frame. This will prevent the wheel from turning, and keep the pedals and sprocket-wheel in position; your fingers may be caught and badly cut if this precaution is not taken. Fasten the small wrench on the little nut, and hold it there with one hand, with the other unscrewing the little screw with a small screw-driver. Should the screw fail to yield easily, a drop or two of kerosene will soften the rust and grit, and help to start it.

Return the nut to the screw end, and place it on the tray. Take hold of one end of the chain, and remove the bar that steadies the rear wheel, then turn one of the pedal cranks, and the chain will come off in your hand. The chain should be placed in kerosene and left to soak.

The enamel of the frame should then be carefully rubbed and polished with canton flannel. A clean piece should be kept for the purpose, for if greasy it gives a dull look to the enamel. The plating should be first polished with a cloth, and then if dull with whiting. Nickel plating takes a beautiful polish with electro-silicon used on canton flannel.

Go carefully over each oil-cup, and be sure it is cleaned, and work around the ends of the axles. Ascertain if either wheel needs adjusting, and look carefully to see that the rims are true. A good way to do this is to hold a pencil-top on the frame against the rim of the wheel, and spin the wheel. If it touches evenly all around, the wheel is true; if uneven, take the bicycle to a repair shop and have the wheels trued as soon as possible.

After cleaning all the bearings, put oil in the oil-cups and replace the chain. It is well to leave the chain soaking in kerosene, and later hang it up to drip, and when dry, it will be found bright and clean; or keep a can of lubricating oil in which to soak the chain, and after draining it thoroughly, wipe clean before replacing on

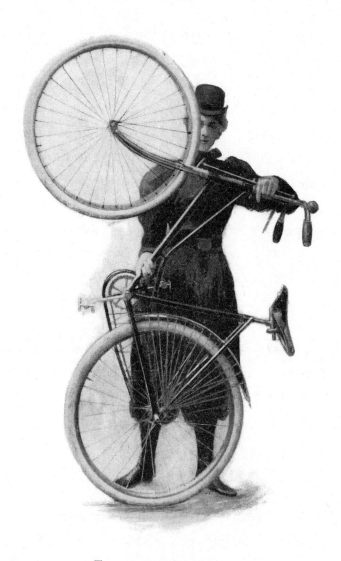

TURNING THE BICYCLE OVER.

the machine. Take an oil-can, and oil each separate rivet. Start the chain on the sprocket, and pull it over the rear sprocket by turning a pedal crank, bringing the ends on the lower side. Place the bar across as before, to keep the sprocket from moving, and then replace the little screw-bolt, using a small wrench, and a screw-driver that fits the screw. Remove the bar, see that the chain is not too tight, and note if it requires any taking up, an adjustment that is done in the rear wheel.

Hold the stick of graphite on a convenient surface of the chain, and turn the cranks; then dust the chain to take off any small lumps of the lubricant, and the wheel is ready to be run. Examine the tires and valves, see that the tires are not too soft, and inflate them. See that the valves are in order, then set the wheel right side up. Replace bell and lantern, rub off any fingermarks, and the bicycle is ready.

If the bicycle has been running for some time, and in spite of the care bestowed on it, the chain runs a little heavy, the pedals don't spin as they should, or the cranks revolve as often as they might, and the wheels are sluggish, there is no remedy but to take down the bicycle, clean it thoroughly, set it up and adjust it. It will require several hours' hard work to do this, combined with a knowledge of machinery and a knowledge of bicycle working, or else enterprise, care, and common sense.

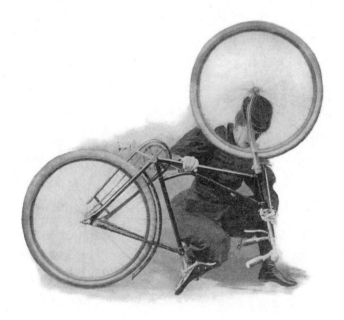

THE BICYCLE TURNED OVER.

Begin work on a wheel perfectly free, as far as the outside can be made so, from sand, mud, and grit. Remove the chain and put it to soak. Have a pan of kerosene, and place each small part in that to soak, and any part that has friction surface or is notably oily or greasy.

Begin serious work on a pedal, which is small and easily handled. If the pedal is a removable one, take it off. If the spindle is stationary, take off the movable parts, first the nuts or screws, then loosen the cones, having a box placed underneath to catch the balls if any should fall out. Support the box well up under the pedal, as the balls bounce and jump about. Even if you have had the pedals off before, and know how it is done, it is well to have something to catch the balls, as otherwise you must atone for any mistake by a scramble. Place the balls in a separate dish of kerosene, and carefully count them. Wipe the movable parts of the pedals with a cloth wet in kerosene, and finish with a dry cloth.

In taking a pedal down, the place of each part should be carefully noted, so that it may be a simple matter to replace the parts. If, the first pedal being now apart, the novice is confused, there is the other pedal to afford comparison. Study that, then return the parts of the dismembered pedal to their proper places, and adjust them. The balls may: prove troublesome; but a screwdriver dipped in Vaseline will pick up any very small balls, and pliers can manage the larger ones. See that cones and washers are replaced, then add a few drops of oil, adjusting the pedal to spin easily without lateral play, and tighten cones and nuts. Spin the pedal for a final test, and then begin on the other pedal.

If after several hours' work, but one pedal is finished, if that one pedal is in perfect order, there is much cause for congratulation. The other pedal may be done very much more easily and rapidly. Of course, it takes time to wipe all the balls and cones, and nuts and screws, and washers and spindles, and when the pedal is in your hand, a little time may be spent to give it an extra rub to brighten its polish. Wipe off any oil that may have shown in the joints of the bearings, and the pedals are finished.

The front wheel should next engage attention. Take a large wrench, and start the bearing cones, and take off the nuts at opposite sides of the ends of the forks. These nuts are screwed on the ends of the axle, and perhaps have metal washers under them. Place them in a box by themselves, and if the forks are notched, there will be nothing to do but to lift out the wheel. If the ends of the forks have only eyes, the forks must be sprung to take the wheel out.

When the wheel is in your hand, avoid letting any grease or oil touch the tire, for it will injure the rubber.

Now proceed to work on the axles. Support the wheel on a large, empty wooden box. The axle is a spindle, and has cones to hold the balls in against the bearings. The cones must be removed and cleaned, and the socket of the hub made clean with an oily cloth followed by a clean one. The axle's spindle should be replaced, and the balls and cones restored to their proper relative positions. Drop in a little oil, adjust and tighten the cones, then spring the wheel back between the forks, and true it; see that it runs even between the forks and that the cones are keyed up firm and even. Replace the nuts, and screw up firm. Wipe off any oil that may have worked out, and spin the wheel to try it. If it runs long and steadily, and has no lateral play, and everything is keyed up tight and true, this part of the work may be considered finished.

Some prefer to use a little pure graphite for the balls, and no oil; and again some bicycles are made without oil-cups. For the first work, oil is safer to handle; but remember that two or three drops are enough. Too much is worse than useless, for oil spreads over a large surface, and will cover all the surface of the bicycle with a thin film, which will need to be constantly wiped off.

The rear wheel may be removed without springing

the frame. Unscrew the adjustment attachment, and the wheel will come out. Clean the rear wheel bearings in the same way you have cleaned those of the front wheel; replace the rear wheel, and put back the adjusting attachment.

Give the crank axle the same care and attention that the wheel axles have received. The pedal cranks are fastened on either end of the crank axle in such a way that the dead centre is avoided as much as possible. The large sprocket-wheel is on the crank axles, and sometimes not movable. The cranks are screwed or fastened with pins to the ends of the axles, and should not be disturbed. Take the large key-wrench from the kit, and start the bearing cones. If the crank must come off, see that the nut on the end of the crank-pin is flush with the end, and place a piece of wood on it before striking it with a hammer, as already explained, to start the bolt or pin. Or if you have some one to help, let a heavy hammer-head be held under the crank beside the bolt, at the other end; and the double shock and recoil from the heavy hammer as the blow is struck will jar the bolt loose.

Remove and clean the cones and balls, then replace and oil them, and adjust the cones tight, ready for adjustment when the cranks are in place. The only bearings left to attend to are those in the head of the frame. Take out the handle-bars, and wipe them and their socket very carefully; never allow any oil to remain there. The handles should never be immovably tight; yet grease, if any were introduced, would perhaps cause them to slip when they should remain in place. The crank axle-key usually fits the cone of the head of the frame, and that may be treated as any other set of ball bearings—loosened, removed, cleaned, replaced, oiled, adjusted, and tightened. Any dust may be removed from inside the frame-head while the bearings are off.

When the head bearings have been restored and the handle-bar replaced, put on the chain and adjust it. The rear wheel is arranged to move forward or back on the frame by the adjusting attachment. This allows the two sprocket-wheels to be placed nearer together or farther apart, and the chain may be stretched and held between them to any desired degree of rigidity or of slackness.

When the bicycle has been set up, the parts correctly replaced, before turning it right side up, go over the entire adjustment of the machine, to see that nothing has been forgotten. Have wrench and screw-driver at hand

and a clean cloth. Begin with the bearings of the front wheel. See that the oil is not working out, and wipe them again. Take the key, and see that they are true and tight. Apply the screw-wrench to the nuts of the fork, and see that they are screwed home. Treat the rear wheel in the same way, and look that both wheels travel on the same line or plane; if they do not, it is because the bearings are out or the frame is bent. Go over the axle bearing, feel the chain, spin the pedals and wheels. A well-adjusted wheel will carry the weight of the valve around quickly and then swing back, showing how sensitive it is to so small a weight. If you are satisfied that everything is right, turn the bicycle right side up, and square the handle-bars. The only way to do this is to stand in front of the bicycle, and take the wheel between the knees while the handles are pulled into place.

The saddle-post and screw-nuts that hold it should be examined and removed and carefully wiped, as well as the socket where they belong. The screw that holds the saddle-post in place does its work by friction, and any oil would prevent it from acting properly, and the saddle would slip. Keep the oilcan carefully wiped, and see that the little spout has a clean round hole at the end that will allow only a drop at a time to escape; for oil travels and spreads in a marvellous manner, appearing where least expected or wanted. If there is a hand-brake on the bicycle, adjusted to alter with the handle-bars, examine it carefully, and wipe the rods. Oil here will allow the coupling to slip and the action of the brake to be impaired.

There are so many things to be carefully observed and accurately done in this kind of work that mistakes and omissions may be easily made by the inexperienced; but there need not be so many blunders, after all, if one works slowly and observingly, taking notes, in writing if necessary, as for instance how far the bearing cones are keyed in when in place, which is the reverse side of the crank and pedal pins, if they are interchangeable, or rights and lefts.

Screw threads are made rights and lefts, and threads are made to fit them in the sockets where they belong. That pedals may not work loose, the spindles are made right and left, with a reverse screw, so that forward pedaling drives them tighter. In the older constructions, the pedal sometimes became unscrewed and fell off, or the nut fell off and the pedal loosened. All such matters should be studied before taking down a machine. Usually the maker's catalogue will describe and illustrate these details. Study that, and learn the names and uses of all the parts of the bicycle, and then you will be prepared to go to work by yourself, or with but little assistance.

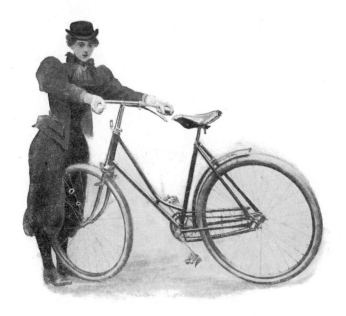

STRAIGHTENING THE HANDLE-BARS.

CHAPTER 16

WHERE TO KEEP A BICYCLE

Almost anywhere that a bicycle can stand or hang will do for a place to keep it; and almost any place will do to go to work on a bicycle—the roadside, the lawn (though the grass is worse than a haystack to lose things in), anywhere, in fact, that may suit your convenience. The accessories of the bicycle should have places where they may always be found, and the bicycle itself should be kept where it will be undisturbed and where it may be kept free from fingermarks, dust, and oil.

With the bicycle should be kept certain conveniences for handling it—a table or bench fitted conveniently, frames to hold the wheel for cleaning and adjusting, a good light to work by, and a place for the tools that are sure to accumulate. There are two kinds of workshop for the amateur—the one that you fit up for yourself, and the one that is fitted up for you. The amateur with a place well fitted out likes to add details of home construction, and the proud owner of a corner cupboard is always anxious to replace makeshifts. In either case, get the best you can, and take care of it. Of tools, the best are always cheapest; but good tools, or tools of any kind, can become a very expensive luxury. Taste for the best comes quickly to even the moderately enthusiastic.

A bicycle rack room should be light, with plenty of head room, and conveniently fitted with racks, shelves, and lockers. Each rack should have its corresponding shelf-room and pigeon-hole, either beside it or above and behind it. There is an infinite variety of racks to select from, from the two stakes driven into the ground or fastened to the floor, to the handsomely finished metal racks with joints to hold the frame at any angle.

If there is but one bicycle to care for, it is better to have its rack and shelf and cupboard together—the rack to hold the bicycle in a proper position, the shelf for sundry attachments, and the cupboard for the lamp and extras. Such a bicycle corner can be made very attractive to look at when everything is arranged and kept in perfect order. When several bicycles are to be cared for together, when neatly set up they make a very pretty showing. If possible, the rack-room should be separate, set apart for that purpose, and kept under lock and key; it should be dry and well lighted, free from frost, and not likely to be over-heated by direct sun-rays in summer. The frost is injurious to metal and enamel; and the sun or too much heat will spoil rubber, and possibly injure enamel as well.

An even temperature, not any special degree of temperature, is requisite; for changes of temperature cause different degrees of expansion and contraction in different materials; and as the steel frame, and the enamel it is covered with, do not expand and contract in quite the some degree, they will gradually work loose from each other, and the enamel will flake or split.

The rubber tire should be kept out of the sun, and the place where it stands should be kept very clean, and no oil allowed about; for oil is injurious to the rubber, and in case of punctures makes repairing very difficult, if not impossible. A rubber surface with even the slightest film of oil will not make a joint, as the oil prevents the rubber surface and that of the cement and the article to be repaired from uniting.

If the workshop is to be used by more than one person, each should have a tool-chest and a work-bench of his own, and each tool-chest provided with lock and key, and each person with a key to the outer door. Tools are but the continuation of the individual brain and will power. What one handles becomes, while in one's hand, a part of one's self, as it were. Tools, therefore, should be individual property always, just as scissors and thimble are, though of course extra tools may be provided for general work. Every one prefers a good pair of scissors to a poor pair, and the same preference is likely to be evinced in the case of other tools. If the tools are common property, the best will be always taken, and often not restored to their proper place.

A bicycle workshop is devoted to metal work, wood-work, and rubber work. The metal work should be kept by itself, and the tools used for metal work only.

The amateur can commence fitting a shop by setting up a small deal table and a vise. The table will do for a work-bench, and one vise will serve for a beginning; it should be of medium size, quite heavy, made of wrought iron or cast steel, and capable of holding a wrench in its jaws, though a less expensive one could be made to do. A cheap vise, however, is pretty sure to break if a strain is put upon it; and, while a good workman could get comparatively good work out of a poor vise, the poor tool in unskilled hands would be sure to show its weak place.

Have a notch cut in the edge of the table to let the vise back to where there is bearing surface; and it is well to have it as far in as convenient, for the weight will thus be supported more steadily. Get a plumber to cut a section of lead pipe about as long as the jaws of the vise, and have the piece of pipe split and flattened. You can do this yourself if you can handle a saw, and have one that is suitable for cutting metal; or a jig saw will do, and the lead can be flattened on a block with a mallet. Screw one of the flattened pieces of lead into the jaws of the vise, leaving about an inch to project above; hammer the projecting part over, and one side of the jaws will have a lead face that can be taken out. Do the same with the other piece of lead. Replace them both, and the vise is fitted with a pair of lead jaw faces, which will be found most useful.

The lead being soft, any small metal object may be held between the jaws without injury, while if the steel face of the vise came in direct contact with the metal, a screw for example, the thread might be bruised; or if the screw were harder than the vise, the face of the jaws would be marred.

With a work-table, a vise, and the bicycle kit, a very fair beginning may be made, and any refractory small part handled with ease. Even the spindle of the axles of one of the wheels may be screwed in, and the bearings removed, while held in this way. The vise will act as a clamp for holding pieces to be polished, and it is most useful in taking a pedal or other small parts down. Above the table should be a tool-rack, three feet of board ten or twelve inches wide, with a ledge or shelf nailed along the lower edge, and a strip of leather or some stiff and pliable material nailed on in loops to hold the tools. Under the table should be kept a couple of boxes—wooden boxes such as canned goods come in will do—one as a receptacle for oil-cans, kerosene, and cloths, and the other to use as a frame. The outfit should be completed by a little bench, and a wooden stool to sit on when working at the table; for much of the work about a bicycle may be done while seated comfortably, and it is always well to save strength when possible.

The ideal room for this purpose should have a good north light, with windows on two sides if possible, and high enough from the floor to allow a work-bench to be placed in front of the window with the light falling upon it, and a space of ten inches or a foot between the lowest part of the window and the bench; this space to be arranged as a rack for tools. The windows should open and shut easily, and be fitted with two kinds of shades, dark green and white, two pairs of shades to each window, two rolling up from the lower part, and two down from the upper part. Nothing is so fatiguing as working by light not suited to the work to be done. With shades arranged in this way, light may be perfectly controlled, and distributed where needed by means of reflectors. Ventilating and heating, also, must be arranged for.

The workshop should have running water, and a closet for working clothes, which are apt to be oily or greasy. There should be plenty of shelf-room, and an extra cupboard or two. The floor should be of wood, unpainted. There should be a bench for carpenter work and carpenter tools; a bench for cabinet-working tools for fine wood-working; a table for rubber and naphtha; and a long, heavy, narrow bench fitted with vises of different sizes and patterns; a table devoted to the blast furnace, a corner for an anvil and portable forge and another for a lathe and power-saw, though these may be dispensed with. The movable furniture may consist of stools and benches of different heights, and the frames necessary to take down and handle a bicycle on.

Metal can be bent, twisted, cut, pressed, elongated, sawed, stretched, and melted into any shape desired. The tools adapted to this work may consist of holding tools, carving tools, molding tools, and bending tools; and contrivances and tools made to perform certain work, as screw-driver, etc.

Cutting tools are knives, saws, files, and chisels, which perform their work by applied power, whether controlled directly by the hand or otherwise.

The metal-working outfit may contain many varieties of tools.

CHAPTER 17

TIRES

In the older forms of wheel, the tire did duty in protecting and strengthening the wheel and holding it together. In the bicycle wheel, the rim is the strengthening and supporting contrivance. The tire protects the rim, and acts as a spring cushion as well, receiving shock and jar. The solid rubber tire was an advance over the old steel tire on the bone-shaking machine, as it was called, in the days when the bicycle was still in its experimental stage.

The solid tire was narrow, and after a certain diameter of material was reached, the weight of rubber became too great if the tire was made larger. It was found that a certain thickness of material was sufficient for wear and tear and that more surface was desired to grip the roadway, and that consequently the tire should be made lighter. Hose-pipe was tried, and did well; and then experiment succeeded experiment in the effort to produce a tire that would fit, wear well, be light, and give speed and resilience.

A pneumatic tire is made of a tough, hard outer material to resist wear, a fibrous inner material to give stiffness and prevent stretching, and an impervious inner layer to retain the air. Rubber is a sticky, gummy substance, easily melted at a comparatively low temperature, and becoming hard when exposed to the air and moderately low temperature; it dissolves readily in benzine or gasoline or naphtha, and is insoluble in water. Grease and oil have a peculiar disintegrating effect on rubber and rubber materials, and are most injurious to them. To prevent rubber substances from adhering to each other, they are prepared in a particular way, and feel dry and gritty to the touch.

Tires are made in layers, and double-tube tires have a separate inner tube of impervious rubber to hold the air, and an outer covering of toughened material, that is quite separate and not necessarily air-tight, to resist wear.

The tire must be held immovable on the rim of the wheel. There is all the pull of the weight of the moving bicycle against the surface over which it moves, and the tire must be secured to the rim in such a way as to keep it forced in place. There are two methods of fastening it permanently to the rim,—with cement or other material of that character, so as to make it a part of the rim, as it were; and by clamping it fast. A cemented tire, or indeed any tire of rubber, should never be left in the sun, as the heat affects the rubber and perhaps the cement.

Changes of temperature affect different materials in different degrees, and the different materials expand and contract, working loose from each other until something gives way, with apparently inexplicable results. When two or more different materials are used in construction in this way, this problem will always present itself.

The tire inflated, the impervious inner covering of the tire tube, which is made of a soft and yielding substance, fills the interstices in the outer covering, rendering it air-tight. Should a hard substance then be introduced into this material, and a puncture occur, it is necessary to locate the puncture. This is very difficult to do if the puncture is small, and the substance that made the hole has been removed. Ascertain first that the trouble is not with the valve of the tire if the air is not retained properly. Then test for puncture in this way. Wet the surface of the tire, and note the bubbles that form under the film of water, and the puncture is found.

The inner surface tire is made to resist the air, and is usually of pure rubber. The outer covering is for strength and wear. Rubber may be repaired with rubber easily enough, and the purer the rubber, the easier it is to cement it with a cement made of pure rubber dissolved in a volatile vehicle. Almost any repair or renovation of the tire may be accomplished with rubber material, rubber cement to be used for plugging, and twine or cotton cloth to be used for strengthening purposes. Small punctures require only plugging from the inside; tears and rents require plugging and reinforcing as well. Each make of tire has its repair-kit and directions for use.

The single-tube tire, with its inner coat, is so made that the inner covering will act as a continuous plug. The soft rubber is compressed, and put on in such a way that the air pressure, even if a puncture occurs, will help to close the hole by pressing on all sides around and about it. To illustrate this principle, cover the outside of the tube with soft rubber cement, and let it dry. Then turn the tube inside out. The rubber will be in an active state of compression. Force air against the surface, and it is easily seen how the rubber is crowded if there is any place made by puncture, and how the hole would be closed.

Numberless punctures are made and resealed, and the tire works all right. The puncture that does not reseal must be plugged or patched. Rubber plugs are made in all sizes; and rubber cement, liquid rubber, is put up in collapsible metal tubes, like paint-tubes, with a pointed spout to introduce the cement behind and through the puncture. There are numberless convenient contrivances made to hold plugs, enlarge holes, and to do the repair work neatly.

In mending a puncture, the tire remains on the wheel, and the work is done from the outside of the tire. If the hole is very small, it must be enlarged sufficiently to introduce the plug. The rubber of the plug is very soft and compressible, and the hole should be considerably smaller than the shank of the plug.

The plug must be held firmly, and forced through the hole, and held in place while the nose of the cement-tube is introduced, and a plentiful supply of liquid rubber smeared over the inside of the hole around and on the plug, and enough extra cement added to flow all about the inside of the tire around the puncture. Pull the plug back by the shank, allowing the head to rest on the inside of the tire, and the shank to come back through the hole. Pull the plug firmly into place by the shank, which should fit the hole very tight. Cut off the projecting end of the plug shank, and the repair is made. Turn the wheel until the plug comes to the lowest point, and keep it there until the cement gets around the plug. To smooth a ragged hole before introducing the plug, when the proper tools are not to be had, a heated wire may be used to make a round smooth hole. Rubber may be handled and cut while wet with water, but must be dry and free from grease to take cement. Always wet the knife-blade before cutting the end off the plug; this will ensure a smooth, clean cut.

A puncture may be repaired by introducing almost any material on the inner surface, and holding it in place; and it is well to know of a few substitutes for the regular repair-kit for emergency use. Punctures difficult to locate may be found by inflating the tire and wetting with soapy water, when a bubble will form where the air escapes.

A puncture that goes all the way through the inner tube of the tire must be repaired on the inside. The outer covering of the tire is porous, and if the hole is plugged or patched on the outside, the air will escape in other directions through the material of the tire. Failing the repair-kit tools, a rubber plug, some liquid cement, a piece of string, and a pair of pliers will do good work. Tie the string to the plug to keep it from slipping, apply plenty of cement to the plug, then grasp it with the pliers, and introduce it through the hole prepared for it in the tire. Pull the string to pull the plug into place, see that there is plenty of cement around and about it, inflate the tire, and the air will hold the plug in place until the cement hardens.

The plugs that are supplied are disks of rubber of different sizes, with stems attached to the centre, and a nice tool is made for the purpose of punching the hole in the tire. When a hole is burned, the charred edges should be removed, and if possible cleaned with benzine. A tire well patched on the inside is almost as good as new, and very serviceable, unless the brake is applied frequently and unevenly, when the plug is almost sure to feel the push.

The commercial patch or plug makes the most satisfactory repair for a puncture, although there are other things that may be used. Rubber bands may be pressed into service, and sheet rubber also may be used. Repair on the roadside is made in the same way as repair in the workshop, the differences being in the conveniences for working and the permanency of the patch. A rent may be repaired with plugs, it being first stitched together, then the plugs introduced, and finally a patch cemented on the outside over the rent to protect the stitches. A puncture may be repaired with rubber bands held in place on a wire, covered with cement, and forced into the hole made in the tire. A piece of wire flattened on the end, a cross piece with a notch cut in it and twisted below, makes a fair repair needle. The end of the projecting rubber cut off, a very fair plug results.

Sheet rubber may be placed over the hole on the inside, though it is difficult to keep it in place. Twisted up and tied into a plug, or spread into place on the inside, the difficulty with this repair is that the patch must be held in place until the cement hardens, and then is liable to work out of place. Inner tube tires are repaired with patches of soft rubber. After the puncture is located, the patch will retain its place by being pressed against the inner surface of the tire when inflated.

To do good work in repairing rubber, always clean the surface of the rubber material thoroughly, washing with benzine when possible; and always test a patch when finished by placing it in water or wetting it, to ascertain that it is satisfactory. On the road a puncture may be plugged in any time under five minutes when located. In the workshop, it is more convenient to hang the wheel up while making a patch, as it is more readily held in place when working from below.

There are many ways of doing makeshift repairs. Melted rosin may replace the rubber cement, and rosin may be found at any tinsmith's. Melt the rosin, and dip the rubber in that to make it stick.

Tire tape may be used in a variety of ways. Find the puncture, cut strips three or four inches long, and place them lengthwise on the tire, lapping the edges at least half way over; then wrap the two thicknesses of tape round and round the tire, and keep lapping the tape each time over the last turn to hold the edge down, making it air-tight. Well put on, tire tape will last for many miles. The tire should be partly inflated while the tape is being put on, and fully inflated when it is all on. Force more air into the tire to cause the tape to grip securely. Such repair, though not permanent, may prove serviceable in emergency.

A simple and effective substitute for the rubber plug is absorbent cotton or jeweller's cotton, well dipped in cement, and the cement worked into the cotton. Quite a large puncture may be repaired with this, and the hole need not be enlarged or burnt to receive it, as the soft mass of cotton fills the irregularities in the puncture. It may be introduced into the puncture either with an ordinary repair tool or a piece of twisted wire. The tire is held on the rim by cement made of shellac or some other equally good cementing substance. Of course, in using a cotton plug, the greatest mass of the cotton should be on the inside of the tire, leaving a stem in the puncture, and then the outside ends should be trimmed off.

The tire may be readily removed with the hands by pulling at right angles with the wheel. Rubber cement may be made by dissolving perfectly pure rubber in naphtha; but the commercial cement is usually found the cheapest in the end.

If you should be so unfortunate as to break down, what are the problems you must meet? The bicycle is made of different materials—iron, metal, steel, wood, rubber, and leather, and each different material requires a different kind of treatment. The general idea in any kind of repairs is to affect the holding of the parts in position with a material that will supply strength and stiffness. The use of glue or cement is merely to hold parts in position, to replace the fractured pieces and keep them in place, to enable the particular part to do its duty, and to keep the piece in place while the cement hardens.

There is room for great ingenuity in handling repair work and in estimating the available resources. The most common accident is a puncture in a pneumatic tire. There are also repairs to be considered to the wooden rims and the spokes and the tubing and lost or broken parts. A great deal of damage could occur in a collision, and the bicycle be in very poor shape, but it can be set right with a little assistance from a mechanic, even though he does not understand the mechanism of a bicycle.

Suppose nothing to be injured except a piece of the supporting tubing; or that the bicycle could be made to go if the rim were spliced or strengthened at a place where it has been split. A temporary repair usually takes considerable time, and should never be attempted unless there is nothing else to be done. A blacksmith shop, unless the smith is very ingenious, is not a very good place to look for assistance; a plumber or tinsmith or locksmith, unless a bicyclist, can help but little. For a broken rim I would betake me to a carpenter shop or carriage maker's. If the break is in a straight piece of tube, get the carpenter to make a round stick, not as long as the broken tube, and fit it to the inside, to slip in easily. Hardware stores keep round wooden rods, and perhaps one of these would answer. Push the round stick up into the tube, and, holding the parts in place, let it slip down into the other part of the break; this will keep the ends of the break together. Then get the carpenter to take two blocks of wood, hollow them out to hold the tube, and screw them fast together, holding the tube between them. If he has an auger-bit the size of the tubing, he can easily bore a hole in a block the size of the tube; then have this block cut in two with the saw, leaving the hole cut in half, and screw the pieces together after they are placed on the broken part. The same kind of a repair may be made on the angles of the frame if the blocks are hollowed to fit. This makes an unsightly job, but can be recommended as strong and safe when properly done.

A broken spoke may be repaired, if it cannot be replaced, by bending the ends of the broken parts into loops; then, taking a piece of wire through both loops, fasten it together, and tighten by screwing it up.

A wooden rim may be whipped or wound. The tire must be deflated first, and removed from the rim at the broken place; then wind fine wire or fish-line about the place, after filling the break with glue or shellac. In wrapping, take care that the turns are made very smooth and even, and close to each other. Then the tire may be cemented and inflated. Of course, there will be a lumpy place on the rim, but it will do until the rim can be replaced.

Any bolt that has lost its nut, when the nut cannot be replaced, may be held by hammering a burr on the end. If the end is too long, a piece may be cut or filed off, and a burr hammered down to hold.

A bicycle cannot travel easily if the frame has been bent out of true; and to straighten a bent frame is an easy matter, Take out wheels, saddle, and handlebars, and use a piece of broom-handle to spring the frame into true; or

CHAPTER 18

MECHANICS OF BICYCLING

All applied mechanical power is the application of lever movement (and lever movement is but the effect of applied power), either simple, compound, or complex.

In the bicycle propelled by human power, we have a series of lever movements, initiated and executed by the highest and most effective mechanism known—the human body, applied human power. There is the seat of power, the point of application, and the object. The bicycle or object is so constructed that it continues the application of power applied.

The lever is described as "a bar or other rigid

instrument having a fixed point for the exercise of power and the application of power to the object to be moved." The series of lever movements in the human body is the most wonderful known.

There are three varieties of levers, of three different degrees of efficiency, known as levers of the first, second, and third classes, or orders, of levers.

In the lever of the first class, the fulcrum is between the weight and the power: P F W.

In the lever of the second class the fulcrum is opposite to the power: P   W.

F

In the lever of the third class the fulcrum is opposite to the weight: P   W.

F

These different powers of levers are used in combination, and produce a great variety of power effects and applications.

Other factors to note are:

That a body in motion persists in maintaining its direction unless other forces intervene.

That the gyroscope overcomes the force of gravity while rapidly revolving.

That a body set in motion tends to move in a straight line.

That the centre of gravity must be maintained by balance if disturbed or shifted.

That force is the cause of a change in the velocity or direction of motion of a body.

That all alterations of velocity take place gradually and continuously.

That centripetal force and centrifugal force are force directed by radial action.

That the air offers resistance, which increases when the air is in motion.

That friction offers resistance to power.

That the smaller the surface presented, the less friction there is to resist.

That resistance must be overcome by power expended for the purpose.

That the base of the bicycle is practically without width, and is usually about from forty-two to forty-four inches long.

That the direction of the base may be changed at will within certain limits.

That the bicycle will fall unless prevented from doing so.

That to prevent a bicycle from falling, or to maintain a bicycle on its base, it is necessary to balance it.

That the constant effort to maintain the bicycle upright upon its base is on account of the motion of the different opposing forces.

The bicycle is constructed to overcome the resisting forces in different ways, supplying as many forces as can be made available to accomplish a particular purpose, permitting a certain choice and discrimination in the matter.

The bicycle has one weight-carrying wheel and a frame and a pivoted wheel. The driving power is applied to the weight-carrying wheel, and the steering is done with the pivoted wheel. The bicycle remains upright because several forces co-operate to enable it to maintain its plane, change direction, and overcome certain resisting and opposing forces.

A bicyclist is propelled at a sufficient velocity to maintain the plane of movement. By altering the centre of gravity, inclining one way or the other, change of direction may be made.

The front or guiding wheel of the bicycle, being controlled by the different angles of resistance it presents to the surface it rotates upon, and not being immovably fixed, can pivot to a plane corresponding to a plane of least resistance. After a little momentum is attained, a bicycle will maintain its speed with but little assistance of power, unless it is accidentally obstructed, or an increase of grade requires an increase of power.

The frame of a bicycle is a compound lever, combining the second and third orders. The wheels are a compound lever of the second and third orders. The fork and handles a lever of the second order.

The forks and handle-bars are set at an angle with the front wheel, thus conveying the touch on the ground or other surface to the pivot head and the hands.

A moving body tends to pursue its direction. A wheel loses its power to change its direction after passing the point of friction. With the forks at this angle, the blow is felt, and change of direction caused by an obstacle conveyed; but the wheel has still some power to maintain its plane from friction, and is steadied by its head. The motion of swaying is conveyed and overcome at the tire base. If the pivot were directly over the tire base, the swing would be given to the wheel; and the tire, having passed its point of friction, would continue to swing. If the head were pivoted on a point, there would be no side friction on the rim; because it is pivoted at an incline, the friction base is increased in proportion, and the wheel, steadied in itself, is easily controlled by an increased line of friction or by prolonging the time from the point of contact.

A body in motion persists in maintaining its plane of motion unless additional forces intervene. The occurrence of these forces is detrimental and frequent, requiring a continuous swing of the guiding wheel either by the hands or by balance. The direction of the base line is continually changed, as it were, broadening the base line. The weight must incline with the front wheel, and the front wheel will support it. If inclined away from the direction of the front wheel, the weight becomes the long arm of the lever, exerting weight against weight at the base of the bicycle, there being no opposing force. The front wheel being turned away, the bicycle falls or slips over.

With the fork at this angle the wheel is inclined, the frame held on the wheel at this angle, as the wheel is turned sideways, it gradually brings the centre directly over the axles, raising the front end of the frame up. This pressure or leverage from the frame tends to keep the wheel straight in the line of least resistance. In turning, the wheel must lift the weight, and push it up; and this factor greatly adds to the steadiness of direction.

A bicycle with the steering wheel held fast will maintain its plane so long as its momentum is not overcome. With the steering wheel the plane of movement may be regained after each opposition, provided the proportionate amount of power is expended.

The radius of a wheel is the long arm of a lever; the pedal crank is the short arm of the lever, though its length may exceed that of the radius of the wheel.

Power and speed are interchangeable. The shorter the arm of the crank, the greater the weight required to balance the long arm at the rim of the wheel (an imaginary line). If the pedal crank is lengthened, it will require less power to move it. At the same time the foot, following the crank, describes a larger circle for the distance travelled by the rear wheel. The crank lengthened, the power is diminished, demanding increased exertion to follow it, the foot travelling at a rate determined by the distance to be traversed.

When the hub rests on the axle of the wheel, there is considerable friction to overcome in the entire length of the hub, the friction, or ability of the wheel to turn, depending on the amount of axle surface. The axle, therefore, becomes heated when the air cannot readily reach the surface to convey away the heat generated by friction.

Weight may be balanced and supported on a point; when weight rests on a sphere, only a point supports weight. By surrounding the axle with balls, the weight is taken from point to point on each ball, and a circulation of air allowed. The weight, carried from ball to ball, gives the advantage of a larger cooling surface in a confined space, while the weight and friction are applied directly to a very limited area. Each ball is also an axle in itself, and carries the weight, and passes it on to the next ball. The balls act as lubricators, preventing the moving surfaces from contact.

The problem of speed produced by power means that speed is obtained at the expense of power expended. The relative size of the sprocket-wheels determines the relative speed of the cranks and rear wheel. To get the greatest speed with the least power possible means diminished friction and lessened weight. The band or chain complies mechanically with these requirements, permitting a certain amount of play, which lessens the danger of sudden strains and jars, and supplies the power to the rear wheel with the least possible loss by friction.

Gear	63	72	76	80
6 ½ crank proportion	4 11–13 to 1	5–13 to 1	5 11–13 to 1	6 2–13 to 1
8 crank proportion	3 15–16 to 1	4 4½ to 1	3 3¾ to 1	5 to 1
6 ½ crank pressure	4.85	5.54	5.85	6.15
8 crank pressure	3.37	3.84	4.5	5.00
8 crank ground covered by large wheel	16 ft.	19 ft.	20 ft.	21 ft.
6 ½ crank ground covered by pedal		40.84 inches		
8 crank ground covered by pedal		50.26 inches		

"*Scientific American Supplement, No. 1025,*" August 24, 1895.

Rating wheel by the amount of progression for each turn of the crank (pedal), the following table, compiled by Henry Starkweather, will be found of advantage:

No. teeth in large sprocket	26-inch wheel. No. teeth in small sprocket.			
	6	7	8	9
18	20 ft	17 ft	15 ft	13 ft
19	21 ft	18 ft	16 ft	14 ft
20	22 ft	19 ft	17 ft	15 ft
	28-inch wheel			
18	22 ft	19 ft	16 ft	14 ft
19	23 ft	20 ft	17 ft	15 ft
20	24 ft	21 ft	18 ft	16 ft

The following table, from the New York *Evening Post,* shows the gear according to the number of teeth on large and small sprocket-wheels:

Sprockets on pedal crank.	28-inch wheel		
	7 sprockets on rear wheel.	8 sprockets on rear wheel.	9 sprockets on rear wheel.
17	68	59 ½	53
18	72	63	56
19	76	66 ½	59
20	80	70	62
21	84	73 ½	65

CHAPTER 19

ADJUSTMENT

In bicycling, the word "adjustment" means much, for the movable parts of the bicycle must be adjusted to suit the requirements of the individual bicyclist, and the mechanical parts of the bicycle's construction adjusted so that they will work together properly.

In a machine properly adjusted, the chain and other gear should run smoothly, the chain be neither too tight nor too loose, and the sprocket-wheels exactly in line. The bicycle wheels should run true and be exactly in line with the frame, and the rear wheel follow the identical plane of the front wheel when in place. The frame should be true and square at all points, and should be examined and tested always after the machine has been travelling by rail or has had a fall. The bearings in all parts of the machine should have their cone-caps in place and so screwed and keyed that the balls run easily without perceptible play. Nuts and washers should all be in place and screwed home. The handle-bar should be tight and square with the front wheel, but only tight enough to turn the wheel on a good surface, not so tight as to prevent it from turning easily if the wheel is caught or held. The proper adjustment for position has to do with the frame, wheel-base, length of crank, height and position of saddle; the curve, width, height, and general adjustment of the handle-bar; the size and number of teeth on the sprocket-wheels, which determines the gear; and the weight, construction, and inflation of the tire.

The saddle is one of the most important, if not the most important, parts of the bicycle to study, as it should provide the fulcrum to work from. Any saddle may be adjusted to be comfortable, but saddles seldom remain comfortable after being adjusted. The saddle should be hard enough to act as a fulcrum and should not give or spring under work, for power is lost on each stroke that presses down on a soft saddle; it should also permit of change of position without readjustment, unless it is intended for racing purposes, for the bicyclist should be able to speed, climb, or coast on a saddle properly constructed for general purposes. Each of these different kinds of bicycle work requires a different application of muscular power, and the saddle should permit of a readjustment of position that will at least accommodate the altered tendency caused by a shifted centre of gravity in grade work.

Every individual is differently proportioned, with differing lever lengths and lever power. If people differently proportioned find the same adjustment possible, it would be for the reason, not that their different requirements average the same, but that the average of their different requirements is the same. A higher gear means greater resistance; a lengthened crank causes the foot to travel in a larger circle while gaining in increased leverage in the lengthened arm.

In determining the proper proportion of crank length and gear, it may be calculated that the same amount of resistance may be overcome by using a higher gear and longer crank as by using a lower gear and shorter crank, the difference being in the rapidity of the stroke necessary to cover a given distance in a certain length of time. This adjustment may be considered equivalent to length of pace and rapidity of pace in walking. It is well to have crank and gear selected by some one sufficiently experienced to make an intelligent choice.

In the lever action of the leg, working the bicycle crank, care should be taken to prevent waste of power in carrying the foot back and behind, rendering the lever movement useless behind the line where the power may be made to tell. This loss will occur when the saddle is placed too far forward. The foot in returning should supply the pull, and lift with a push-back. The power here gained cannot compensate for power lost on the forward and down thrust, and the saddle should be placed far enough back to permit of the full power of the forward push and downward thrust. The knee should never fully extend when the pedal is pushed to the point where it is furthest from you, for if it is, there is danger in hill-climbing of straining the knee as well as the tendons and muscles of the back of the leg.

The handle-bars should be adapted to the work to be done, whether racing, touring, or ordinary. They certainly should not be high enough to prevent them from taking part of the weight of the body, nor so low as to cramp any portion of the trunk.

Fatigue, with its various manifestations, cramp, stiffness, and numbness, comes from too long a period of work without change of position. For this reason different muscular combinations should be called to do the same work, or different work should be done with unused muscular combinations, permitting rest or partial rest to muscles that have been taxed.

A bicycle should be fitted with adjustable handle-bar and saddle-post, and in case of fatigue or cramp, a slight change in the adjustment will reduce the tendency at once. Travelling should be done with as little weight on the saddle as possible, working on the pedals and resting on the handles. But when it comes to climbing, the push must be located from a fulcrum, and that fulcrum must be the saddle. All weight must be removed from the handles, and the wheel ridden by balance.

A hill should be coasted with the weight all on the saddle, the feet supported, and the handles held firmly and lightly, a proper average position for continuous work being, however, maintained. To carry weight forward, the weight should be forward of the centre of gravity, and the hands dropped.

The question of handle-bars, with the reason of their many varying curves, may pertinently be discussed here. The bar is a pair of levers finding a common fulcrum in the head or centre bar, and the difference in curve has to do with the distribution of weight and the touch best suited to control the bicycle according to position and individual balance and lever power. A distribution of weight and leverage may be made without altering the wheel base by the use of a different pattern of bar that seems to suit the individual touch.

To analyze the curves in a handle-bar, and their different lever values, would be difficult. Preference has much to do with it, and this may be accounted for by the different steering touch of the differently adjusted bars. The forward drop should never be so great that the face cannot be lifted easily and the eyes always able to see up and ahead.

In the tire we look for elasticity, and the amount of air it contains has much to do with the comfort of the rider and the speed of the wheel. Soft tires are adapted for a rough or stony road. The soft tire may wear out a little sooner, but the extra wear is fully compensated by the gain in lessened shock and apparent improvement of wheeling surface. A very hard tire is not necessarily made of rubber. The advantage of the rubber tire is its elasticity, which should come between the fulcrum and the power.

To attain a proper position and its equivalent adjustment, first have the saddle as nearly right as possible so that you can work comfortably; then have the handles and the height of the bar tested, working on these until you can determine if the saddle is too far forward or too far back. Then change the height of the bars to suit the saddle.

Next attend to gear. Find if with comfort you could exert more pressure on the pedals. If so, have the gear increased. If there is cramp in the foot, or the foot feels strained, have the length of crank changed. If the foot is long in proportion to the other lever lengths, lengthen the crank to permit of freer instep play; or have it shortened to relieve a strained feeling in the foot. The crank length may be changed to relieve either cramp or strain in the leg and thigh until the pressure and length are arranged to suit the natural step or pace.

While these adjustments are in progress—and it may take months to determine them—the shoe may cause discomfort. The slightest pressure, a shoe too tight or ill-fitting, would be responsible for much more discomfort than could possibly be caused by either crank or gear. Waist-bands, or any pressure on the trunk, will cause numbness of the foot; and a saddle of imperfect construction or wrong adjustment would be responsible for the same evils—unequal pressure and unequal strains and overcharged blood-vessels, with their accompanying discomforts of cramp, fatigue, numbness, and more permanent disorders.

CHAPTER 20

EXERCISE

How shall be determined the proper amount of exercise for any individual? The human body is constructed for use, and will suffer from want of use, rust out, as it were; and it will suffer from over-use if any one set of muscles or any one supply of nerve power is overtaxed.

Exercise, in some form, is necessary for every one; work is necessary; recreation is necessary. Rest is to recreate, to renew. The food that we eat is digested and made into blood; the blood flows through the system of tissues, depositing building material and taking up waste matter. The arterial system, physiologists tell us, supplies the new material; the venous system takes up the waste material, returning the blood to the heart, after which the fresh air comes in contact with the blood in the lungs, and is aerated and oxygenated, and waste material given off. The heart pumps the blood through the arterial and venous systems. When we move or work, more blood is needed, and the heart pumps harder. When little or no exercise is taken, the heart loses its vigor from want of use; and it may be strained if overtaxed.

Brain power and nerve power depend on the blood supply for renewal of their tissue. Any organ or any combination of organs and muscles, when exercised, give off their accumulated material, and then, after a limit of assimilation is reached, the products are reabsorbed. The materials properly accumulate only when needed.

These facts bring to our notice three conditions—a condition of atrophy, or too little use; a perfect condition of equilibrium of forces; and a condition of strain from over-work. In the condition of equilibrium or perfect health, the brain is active and the muscular tissue under perfect control. The mind can receive impressions, and can convey them at will; and the muscles obey without difficulty and without fatigue, because of the great existing power of resistance. On the power to resist fatigue depends the power of prolonging exertion.

In exercising we exert our powers, and if from lack of use or other cause our amount of stored energy is small, exercise for even a very short period will produce a condition which makes rest absolutely necessary. Muscles must be gradually accustomed to work; and if work is prolonged beyond the point where exercise is beneficial, a state of tension and exhaustion ensues which can be remedied only by rest prolonged enough to allow the system to recuperate. Where the tissues, from disuse, have come to have little resistance value, a very gradual and persistent course of exercise must be determined upon, for unaccustomed muscles are quickly fatigued, and the subsequent rest they require may seem out of proportion to the work done. This condition of affairs is discouraging when not understood; yet there can be no different result except in degree; and in degree must the condition be changed and the tissues gradually renewed. If there is but little power stored, only little may be used until the power of assimilation is established.

The thin woman is benefited by bicycling; the liver works better, the food digests better. The stout woman is benefited, for the exercise hardens and condenses the flesh. The average healthy woman is kept in the best of health by the exercise and plenty of pure, fresh air. For the sedentary, the undeveloped, and the insufficiently nourished, the bicycle seems to work wonders. All the powers are accelerated and a general renewing of tissues takes place. The organs of digestion are stimulated and do better work, the appetite improves, the complexion brightens, and the mind responds readily. But people of either of these classes should be careful not to prolong exercise until loss of appetite is brought about; for the exercise should tend to increase, not to decrease, the desire for food and power of assimilation.

Baths should be taken in moderation, the skin being kept in free, healthy condition by dry rubs and tepid baths until the system is brought to the state where the cold bath can be used beneficially. The diet should be generous and wholesome, and care should be taken to avoid food that does not digest easily. Sufficient clothing should be worn but not too much, and all exercise should be avoided that might produce very copious perspiration. Only a healthy activity of the skin should be induced, and plenty of water drunk.

Do not work nervously. Go to work gently, and save your energies to make the wheels go around. A thin person can remain thin and a fat person remain fat while exercising assiduously if the exercise is not properly directed.

To overcome fat, persistent, systematic, and regular exercise is needed, and attention to diet must be considered essential. For the food consumed produces certain results; and if the system selects and digests most readily the fat-producing elements, their amount should be curtailed, and a diet of good working quality chosen. Fat is burned in producing heat; but if the same amount of fat-producing elements are again taken into the system, the same amount of fat results. The fat-producing tendency must be overcome, and the fat already accumulated consumed, until a good healthy average of tissue is produced and maintained.

Tea and coffee are not foods; they retard the assimilation of tissue, and must be eliminated from the diet of the weight-reducer. Sugar and starch—the latter when eaten is converted into sugar—are heat-producing foods, first forming fats which are used as energy-producing material. Persons wishing to reduce weight, therefore, must manufacture, not so much fat, but bone and sinew. To produce these, nitrogenous foods must be eaten. Fat consists largely of water; and heavy work, like hill-climbing, which induces free perspiration, is desirable. But any one wishing to seriously undertake weight-reduction should learn to enjoy bicycling for itself before attempting this application of the exercise.

Excess of fat produces physical laziness, which is hard to overcome; and stout persons, after exercise, crave fat-producing elements of food to reduce the tissue consumed. A taste seems to develop for sweet stuff and mild stimulants, and it is difficult to refrain from indulging it. Stout people are apt to believe, also, that they cannot endure exercise. They cannot comfortably, and must work with care until they are in a fair state of balance, where exercise ceases to fatigue, before attempting anything like scientific weight-reducing. Sufficient exercise regularly taken, proper diet persistently selected, will finally have the desired effect.

Exercise sufficiently to produce good, thorough perspiration; take a bath and rub down, and put on fresh clothing; avoid tea and coffee, sugar and ice cream, dessert and pastry.

For those in health and in the habit of exercising regularly, there are only the dangers of the sport to avoid while enjoying its pleasures and benefits.

CHAPTER 21

TRAINING

If you intend a fifty-mile or a week's trip awheel, it will be very necessary to accustom yourself to the work before attempting a distance you have not yet covered. Suppose, though your muscles are unaccustomed to long-continued exercise, that you know how to wheel a bicycle and are anxious to go with your friends. They perhaps wheel for an hour or two hours daily, or for several hours twice a week. They are afraid to take you with them; and you feel sure that you can go as far as they do, and at the same rate of speed.

You must make your opportunity and prove your ability. Suppose you can wheel for half an hour without fatigue. Wheel that half-hour every day the weather permits; know your distance and your road; and then practise increasing speed, that is, do your distance in less than the half-hour without hurry. Start slowly, and keep the pace until you get your breathing apparatus steady; then ride faster, and maintain that pace; and so on, in increasing ratio. If you have been in the habit of covering your distance in five minutes under the half-hour, next time add that distance to your spin, and do it in your limit time. When you easily do five miles in half an hour on the road, add a mile or more for the next two or three spins; then do not wheel for one day; the next day wheel twice the distance, wheel eight miles, and rest a day. Then double your distance again. If you cannot do this without feeling the effects seriously, go back to where you made your greatest distance with ease, and start from that point again.

Keep a careful record of your outings, dates, wind, sun, time of day, and humidity. The latter is very important, for on a hot, dry day, greater distance can be done with safety than when evaporation is slow. Consider all the conditions when you find that you are fatigued, and decide if the trouble is with yourself or with the weather. Do not start for at least an hour after eating, and always rest after exercise before taking a meal. Observing these directions, you will soon find that you are making very fair progress, that your confidence is assured, and that you have acquired a certain amount of endurance, and can attempt any reasonable distance.

Exercise transforms, making the inactive capable of performing work and of enjoying opportunities for using their newly discovered powers. The weak are strengthened; the strong retain and renew their stores of strengthened; the young are symmetrically developed, and the older remain supple and active. Exercise preserves and develops all parts of the organism that are capable of performing work. Exercise is work, muscular work; and in working the muscles, all the tissues become readjusted, and all materials and accumulations tending to hinder movement are diminished in quantity and equalized in distribution.

Ease of movement and a state of muscular inactivity are incompatible. To be active, one must work; and the whole organism will respond, and adjust itself to the conditions imposed by occupation and manner of living. The complicated mechanisms and intricate processes of the human body adapt themselves to required conditions; it is only necessary to determine what those conditions shall be to produce certain results.

It is difficult for some to overcome the tendency to a state of inactivity; and there are others to whom even the contemplation of repose is distasteful. The physiological effects produced by exercise differ in different individuals, active persons and those not in the habit of doing muscular work being very differently affected. For exercise, of whatever kind, is muscular work, and "muscular work tends to modify the nutrition of all motor organs and to give them a structure favorable for the performance of work."

All muscular work is done through the contractile power of the muscles. By use the fibres become freed from fat and other accumulations, the muscles increase in size, the contractile power becomes greater, and the impedimenta of fat, etc., are removed by the processes that are accelerated by movement. "Repose causes atrophy of muscular tissue," and the necessary discernment and powers of discrimination must be cultivated to avoid a tendency either in the direction of over-doing or of insufficient exercise.

"The effect of muscular exercise is to render vital

combustion more active; it causes more active processes of assimilation." "Muscular education leads to an economy of forces. Practice leads to a diminution of muscular expenditure"—more work done for power expended. For the power to perform work depends on knowing how to do it properly. Real strength lies, not so much in the mass of muscular tissue as in the ability to use it.

"Exercise of strength demands the simultaneous action of a great number of muscles." "Exercise of speed involves repetition of movement and the application of nervous energy." "Exercises of endurance permit of economy of fatigue," and are characterized by the necessity of perfect equilibrium between muscular effort and the powers of assimilation of the system.

In exercise of strength, every muscle should bring its whole force into play, and the bony structure is united by pressure to make a rigid whole. "Exercises of speed are accompanied by fatigue out of proportion to the mechanical work represented." "Every movement needs the intervention of a great number of muscles; each muscle must contract with definite force in order that the whole work may lead to definite movement."

Co-ordination is the operation of choosing the

muscles which shall participate in a certain movement and of regulating the exact quantity of nervous energy necessary to produce the right amount of contraction. Automatism is acquired by practice; and the muscles must be exercised regularly to enable them to respond intuitively. A complicated series of movement can only be acquired gradually, unless the mind has a large number of muscular combinations at command.

"Exhaustion will result from overwork even when well fed." "Exercises of endurance do not disturb the working of the organs; while increasing their activity, it gives to the system the power to repair wasted tissue, even during work." Carbonic acid is not formed in excess, and is eliminated without producing noticeable results.

The bicyclist, even though indulging moderately in the pastime, must consider these things, and determine the course to be pursued; otherwise the exercise will prove a bane instead of a blessing. There are principles capable of general or special application; and there are special laws that may be generalized; and all may be made to accord with the exercise of bicycling, but each individual must accept a certain responsibility in the matter. The bicycle having been accepted as a means, the end sought for can be attained only by its intelligent use and application.

One of the many advantages of cycling is that the exercise involved is not limited to the use of any one set of muscles. The legs propel the machine, the muscles of the trunk engage in balancing the body, and the arms are employed in steering and controlling the front wheel. All the larger joints are active, and are made supple as well as strengthened and developed. Muscles, unless directed by mental effort, are useless. The bones give stiffness, and act as levers and fulcrums; the muscles are tools of the mind, levers wherewith to pull and push the bones into position.

Precision of movement means economy of expenditure of force, no more effort being expended than is necessary for the act of the moment. People who hunt for the pedal, and try for the saddle two or three times, and fall off because the bicycle fails to start, work hard enough to have mounted a number of times; that is, they have lifted or supported their own weight in different directions a number of times without attaining their object. They appear to be awkward; they are really unaccustomed to their work. Practice will accustom the muscles to the work they have to do.

Try to do one thing only at a time. If it is mounting, for instance, memorize each thing that must be done; how, when, and where to do it. Do not think, because the mind does not at once grasp all that is forced upon its attention, that your brain is of inferior quality; it may not be able to adapt itself to that particular mental process at that minute. But the effort made will result in added tissue, and next time there will be more hope of success. Increase by a little at a time the amount of exercise undertaken. You can gauge the practice you need only by the amount of attention you give to the subject. After muscles are once trained to an exercise, the mind will not readily lose power to reproduce the combination, and experience begins to help.

Endurance means well-directed strength as well as capacity of power stored in reserve; and the aim of all athletic work is to give an increased store of strength, vitality, and power to draw upon, not merely to expend the stock already on hand.

The muscular development that comes with bicycle exercise will often cause surprise. In persons unaccustomed to active exercise, the increase is most noticeable on the chest and forearms, the chest development increasing two and three inches, the arm and forearm in proportion, and the whole muscular system gaining in firmness and tone. Persistent bicycling, prolonged exercise on the wheel, speed work on the track, develop disproportionately the muscle of the leg. The track-man, therefore, prepares for his season of work, not by exercising and developing his legs, but by general exercise and special work that will develop the arms and back and other sets of muscles not called upon for heavy work during the season when he is to do his best. Getting up speed, increasing speed, and hill-climbing all tend to develop the muscles of the leg, which in such exercise are called upon for the heavy work of push and thrust, using a concentrated power to propel. Light dumbbell work is recommended as a good alternate for bicycle work and a means of keeping the muscular system in balance.

Leisure and the weather limit bicycling; other causes are incidental. The weather, indeed, affects bicycling more than any other sport. One of the most imperative needs of bicycling is rapid evaporation, and conditions that do not permit of that are unfavorable. Observe atmospheric conditions, therefore, and avoid severe work when the dew point is approached.

All the hard work wanted can be accomplished in half an hour after the wheel has been taken out; or it may be used as a vehicle for travelling steadily hour after hour for days consecutively; or an invigorating spin of two or three hours may be taken, regulating the pace and the work. One of the things to know about a bicycle is that you can get almost any kind of work you want out of it. To realize that you are doing the work you have been accustomed to have a horse do for you, and in a similar way, and to know that many of a horseman's rules for the care of their working animals may be equally well applied to human beings who do the same work, is apt, perhaps, to cause a sensation of unpleasant surprise. It is a fact, however, that there is much information about the care of horses that the cyclist may study and apply with advantage.

The bicycle is not an iron horse; it is more like skates; is in some things like a boat; in some like a coasting sled; and in many ways is different from anything else. It seems alive at times, as does a boat; but it is the power propelling it that causes the delusion. The only thing alive about bicycles is the persons who propel them; and if they are only half alive before attempting to mount, they will become very alert and keenly appreciative of all that concerns them long before the sport has ceased to be a novelty.

"Exercise is important as a regulator of nutrition." "The best athletic exercise for increasing the size of the chest is that which compels the deepest inspiration." The lower limbs, with their masses of muscular tissue, are most capable of awakening the respiratory need which is proportioned to the expenditure of force. Exercise induces change of shape as well as change of size; and too much exercise of any one kind will produce a local effect.

Breathlessness is not the only form of fatigue, and fats are not the only reserve material. Nitrogenous products of combustion, which cannot be derived from fatty substances, are produced by work; and these are stored among the reserve material, and produce stiffness, as fat produces breathlessness.

In no other sport is the blood sent coursing through the veins in the same way as in bicycling; and as there is not a very great quantity of that wonderful fluid passing and repassing through the circulatory system, any obstruction or pressure is instantly felt and provided for. To avoid giving nature unnecessary trouble in providing for interrupted or unequal circulation, not even a glove that is the least tight should be worn; indeed, the covering of head, hands, and feet should be carefully selected. And the same precaution should be exercised with regard to all clothing. No tight underwear should be worn, and nothing like equestrian tights, which interfere with surface circulation. The waist and lower ribs must be kept free. You should never ride so hard as to allow the air to force the ribs out and in, so that you cannot control them. It is a good rule not to ride so hard that you cannot hold your breath at pleasure.

It is important always to remove perspiration before cooling; therefore, take a bath at once on coming in from a ride; if you cannot do that, rub off with a dry towel, or sponge with tepid water, and rub dry gently; then put on dry underclothing. The cold bath is most invigorating and refreshing, and never more refreshing than after bicycle exercise; but all cannot use it with good results. Provide for your change of underclothing before starting out, and if you do not intend to return, take it with you.

Remember always that it is essential to provide an entire covering for the body that will admit of free exhalations, and warm enough to prevent chilling under all circumstances. While riding, provided the condensing moisture is allowed to escape, it is quite possible to feel overheated, yet the skin must be protected from chill resulting from rapid motion through the air. Air pressure and evaporation nearly balance each other, and the extra heat caused by exertion is tempered by moisture and the constant fanning of rapid locomotion. These effects are most appreciably felt upon halting. If the covering is thin, of light weight, and of too hard a texture to admit of quick passage of air and steam, the garments at once become saturated with moisture, and a serious chilling follows. Even if the halt be but short, it will be found that an appreciable time passes after remounting before one becomes warm, and the distaste for work that follows is a sure indication that something is amiss. If energy were preserved, instead of wasted in warming up after halting, the benefit of the rest would be felt.

A proper porous material should be always worn. With a flannel shirt-waist and woollen sweater, even in quite warm weather, riding is not at all uncomfortable; but substitute a Holland linen coat for the sweater, and the rider will be first very warm, and then very damp indeed and most uncomfortable. Nature provides various means for keeping the body at an even temperature, and it is most essential not to disturb this balance. While working, heat is generated, the skin becomes moist, and a normal temperature is maintained by the rapid evaporation. Too little covering means too great evaporation and lowering of temperature; and even if no chill is experienced, the too rapid cooling invents good working results, and stiffness is apt to set in with fatigue after the day's work, and a languid, sleepy feeling on the day following.

Too much stress cannot be laid on the necessity of being able easily and expeditiously to adjust or redistribute the clothing. Flannel is a good nonconductor of heat, but the bicyclist must use discrimination in selection. Too heavy flannel will induce a copious and weakening perspiration; insufficient clothing will allow the body to be chilled by too rapid evaporation.

One of the greatest benefits to be derived from bicycle exercise is the free, healthy action of the skin that is induced. If this activity is retarded by pressure, much injury may be done by the holding and reabsorbing of waste matter. This reabsorbed matter, which is a direct poison and must be worked off again in the complexities of the system, causes languor and headache and a feeling that exercise is of no benefit, as indeed it is not if proper hygienic laws are not complied with.

While in the open air, there is little danger to be apprehended from damp clothing, as oxidation is going on freely. It is under shelter that danger lurks, where the air does not circulate freely. The underwear should be changed before eating, or the food will do little good. Where you can get shelter, you can usually find conveniences for making the change; otherwise, it is better to eat in the open air.

Digestion involves muscular action as well as chemical processes. Wherever in the system muscular work is being done, the blood is needed in large quantity to enable the muscular processes to continue. In the process of digestion important chemical work is accomplished by the action of certain juices or secretions of the stomach, and rhythmical muscular work in the walls and coatings of the stomach is required to regulate their supply. It may be easily understood, therefore, that digestion should be properly or rather uninterruptedly accomplished, and it cannot be thus properly accomplished if too much of the blood supply is called away in the earlier stages of assimilation.

Active muscular work should never be undertaken immediately after a full meal. The more food there is to be digested, the more work there is to be done, the less capable is the rest of the system for severe work. Such work, after eating heavily, would involve an interruption, almost a suspension, of digestive processes, and a consequent difficulty in the adjustment of the processes involved in muscular work. It would mean a much longer time to get the second wind, inability to do hard or heavy work, as well as inability to prolong the work without discomfort. Such a course of action must lead to serious complications and derangements of the digestive functions and eventually induce liability to disease.

It is very injurious, also, to attempt to perform heavy work fasting, or to prolong the period of exercise when food or rest is required. The human machine requires a certain amount of fuel, and the supply must be taken at regular intervals, or reserved material, which is too valuable to be recklessly expended, will be consumed.

A mixed diet, with plenty of variety, is the best to work on, everything to be thoroughly cooked. Three good meals a day, and no eating between meals; though, when tired, it is not well to work on an empty stomach, and if you are delayed it is better to eat something while waiting than to go too long without eating. Beef and mutton are always good food; and fresh vegetables, fruit, milk and eggs, and cereals either with cream and sugar or milk and sugar. Simple desserts are not harmful, neither are they necessary.

The so-called sustaining power of stimulants merely enables one to burn up reserve tissue, to use up more fuel, to produce more power. Work done under such conditions is forced work, like the forced draught of a steam-engine using power to force the air into the furnace. In both cases, intense heat and great power can be produced, and corresponding radiation and depression occur while the system is undergoing its processes of restoration. Tea, coffee, bouillon, are stimulating, and good as food accessories; but they are not good to work on.

CHAPTER 22

BREATHLESSNESS; THE LIMIT MECHANICAL

Seated awheel, the bicyclist feels master of the situation. The bicycle obeys the slightest impulse, moving at will, almost without conscious effort, virtually as much a part of the rider, and as easily under control, as hand or foot. It is because weight is supported and friction overcome that the bicyclist loses consciousness of effort as he moves, with seemingly no limit to endurance.

A trouble often experienced is breathlessness. For this there are several causes. Sometimes the machine is started too hurriedly and before the processes of the body have had time to adjust themselves. To work easily, the muscles must be heated gradually, until they are brought to the proper point of tension. Again, the easy movement of the wheel often causes the cyclist to become oblivious of the fact that the muscles are working quickly while doing easy work, that the power applied is being converted into speed with little appreciable effort, until suddenly his breath becomes labored, and a halt must be made for rest. We need not attempt here to give the figures for power expended and work done, though both factors may be estimated.

Technically, effort is a physiological condition involving complicated chemical changes and concentration of power. The work of the lungs is done mechanically, automatically, is muscular work, involving chemical changes and giving chemical results. We breathe in air full of oxygen; we exhale air loaded with carbonic acid. Muscular effort produces carbonic acid through chemical changes in the tissues of the body. The oxygen of the air, taken into the lungs to purify the blood, is absorbed and stored. Easy muscular movements give off a limited quantity of carbonic acid and other products, but not more than can be eliminated without readjustment of processes. When a succession of efforts is made, involving the manufacture of larger quantities of carbonic acid, the eliminating capacity is correspondingly taxed.

In making an effort, the lungs become momentarily fixed, and their regular respiratory movement is suspended. Carbonic acid is held, not given off, and a feeling of suffocation is observed. Unless respiration is restored by a pause, poisoning by the waste products ensues, they being reabsorbed, and inducing discomfort and fatigue. Working with effort, the lungs should be free to expand and contract. To this end it is all-important to exhale, expelling the air from the lungs by compression of the chest after severe exertion. Air rushes naturally into the chest cavity; attention, therefore, should be directed, not to getting in air, but to expelling the air already in the lungs. This successfully done assists materially in bringing about that desirable condition known as "second wind," and gives control over the muscles of the chest, which enables waste products to be readily eliminated.

"The intensity of breathlessness during exercise is in direct proportion to the expenditure of force demanded by the exercise in a given time." Breathlessness is due to power expended in a limited time. This, at least, is one of the inducing causes. On the bicycle, power is converted into speed. In hill-climbing, shortness of wind is due not so much to position on the wheel as to the amount of power expended in doing the work. If power is wasted, the work attempted is usually not accomplished; if intelligently expended, the work is done easily and well, leaving the bicyclist in condition to renew the effort when necessary.

Hill-climbing is like stair-climbing; power is expended in a succession of efforts made in raising the weight on an ascending plane. The weight must be lifted, either pushed up or pulled up, and the respiratory need is increased. The hill-climber must aim to mount with as little effort as possible and to make the ascent with the minimum expenditure of power.

Rapidly increased heart-beat is accompanied by deeply inflated lungs and a tendency the bicyclist should guard against to work open-mouthed. Here the question of tight clothing comes prominently forward. Sitting erect and holding by the handlebars, the bicyclist's upper chest muscles are held comparatively fixed or rigid; the arms, being used for support, act as levers holding down the upward expansion of the chest. The air, being compressed, is forced laterally and downward. The downward expansion of the chest is checked by the movement of pedaling, there being a constant upward pressure in the ascending stroke and an increased muscular compression in the descending stroke. With a tight belt, the breathing is chiefly upward, and downward when sitting or walking, the lateral expansion depending on the width and compression of the belt.

When working on a bicycle, with the hands fixed and holding hard, the upper chest is comparatively rigid, the muscles below the diaphragm hard at work; and muscles at work do not admit of compression, which prevents the diaphragm from moving downward. The diaphragm is a muscular wall, stretched across the trunk below the lung cavity and near the waist-line. If the lower muscles of the trunk are actively at work, the diaphragm can be distended but a little way in a downward direction by lung pressure. The air in the lungs, which are hard at work, and over-full, presses against the heart, and makes harder work for that organ. When the lungs are distended, any clothing that can be felt about the waist exerts more or less pressure. The lungs of a bicyclist at work are constantly distended, seldom deflated, and an equal pressure is exerted in all directions. The diaphragm is forced downward, pressure comes on the large blood-vessels, and the legs feel tired as one of the results of the constriction. Pressure on the heart and the large blood vessels of the lung cavity causes rush of blood to the head and gives a heated look to the face and a feeling of faintness and headache.

The muscles of the waist are elastic, but lose their elasticity when not in use. Fat accumulates, and is pressed down, usually below the belt, causing the muscles of the figure to sag and the trunk to lose its proper lines. Compression of the waist while cycling is dangerous, and will cause enlargement of the hips and distort the lines of the figure below and above the waist. If tight clothing must be worn, do not wear it while exercising any more than while sleeping.

Bicycling is a great equalizer of tissue. The system, when this exercise is moderately indulged, is freshened as is a city by a heavy rain, all accumulations and deposits being swept away.

There is a difference, a very great difference, between muscular fatigue and breathlessness, and the two conditions should not be confused. Breathlessness is general fatigue; muscular fatigue is fatigue localized. When you are breathless, all your muscles are tired; they do not want to work and are indeed incapable of performing work.

Work performed by the lower limbs causes breathlessness more quickly than any other kind of exertion, and the bicyclist must bear this fact in mind. The respiratory need is increased in proportion to the amount of carbonic acid in the blood. The lower limbs can perform a great deal of work in a few seconds, the large masses of muscle in the legs at work throwing large quantities of carbonic acid into the blood to be given off or eliminated by the lungs.

Each individual has his own limit or pace, at which he can do work most easily. If this pace is exceeded, effort follows and increased expenditure of power; a greater quantity of carbonic acid is produced to be given off; and fatigue is induced sooner than when working at the pace which can be kept without extraordinary exertion. Every bicyclist knows his own natural pace, and when departing from that must expect to be winded sooner or later.

Rapid work on the bicycle is similar, as muscular exertion, to running, racing, speeding, and sprinting. Here we have the time limit,—great speed produced in a short time; tissue consumed, and carbonic acid produced in large quantities to be quickly eliminated. Increased effort means more power expended. The fixed lung cavity means lessened capacity for increased air-consumption and greatly lessened means of inhaling and expelling air. One of the effects produced by carbonic acid in the blood is a stimulation to increased effort, which causes a desire to prolong work after reasonable limits have been exceeded, a feeling that more must be done, rather than a desire to stop and rest.

Second wind is the condition produced by the adjustment of the processes of the body to the new state of exertion, where the heart and lungs balance and work according to the demands of the new condition. A pendulum, slipped on its spindle and let go, swings irregularly until it finds its new rhythm. The rhythm that corresponds with its weight, momentum and length of spindle, leverage, is the rhythm of the work. All repeated work has a rhythm, and the movement disturbed requires a little time for readjustment. The heart and lungs work automatically and rhythmically, and any new movement disturbs their rhythm, which must be adjusted for change of occupation or exercise until the balance of the working functions is established.

The second wind usually comes after the first fifteen minutes of work. Quickly acquired, it means rapid and easy adjustment of processes, a quick response to effort, and little power wasted. Though individuals differ in this respect, a difficulty in getting the second wind, when exercise has been suspended for a time, will sometimes be experienced, and care should be taken not to overwork when taking up an exercise that has been for some time discontinued.

When you have had exercise enough, stop and rest. Change of occupation, turning from active mental work to active muscular work, has been said to give rest to the mental faculties. Though they perhaps do, in a sense, experience rest, it might be unwise to assert that this rest is really recuperative. Repeated alternation from active mental exercise to active physical exercise would inevitably result in a state of exhaustion, in which the reserve fund of energy or strength would be completely consumed. It is a more accurate statement that a certain amount of muscular work, which will restore the balance of the system, is a good preparation for rest after active mental exertion.

During mental work of any kind, muscular work must be performed; for breathing, seeing, moving the hands, require muscular movement. The question, therefore, resolves itself into one of degree of work done and equilibrium of forces to be maintained, rather than one of restoration of one set of faculties by the overtaxing of another set. Good muscular work cannot be accomplished without the exercise of brain and will; therefore, when the mind is actively employed, a certain amount of muscular tissue is consumed, though not enough to maintain the system in a state of bodily activity. For body and mind, to be in a state of perfect health or equilibrium, should be equally active.

The tissues of the body are constantly renewed, and the amount of work, mental or muscular, that can be accomplished is determined by these constantly renewing processes. The amount of material taken up and stored for use depends upon the amount of material needed; and this is gauged by the amount of work already done, and restricted by the amount of work the material is capable of performing. The balance of work and rest, quantity and quality, varies with different temperaments.

Training means nothing more than preparation. For those engaged in active mental occupation it is well to consider if they are giving themselves the best preparation for resisting the fatigue consequent upon their occupation. Cycling is a pastime and sport, and may be a relaxation and the alternate of other athletic exercises. After the machine is under control, the muscular work becomes virtually automatic; and for this reason cycling, in its various forms, has proved so beneficial as a relaxation.

Overwork produces the effect of poisoning of the system, and reduces its power of resistance. This poisoning is produced by the waste products of the system, which accumulate during work, as the forces for eliminating them are overtaxed; and before work can be properly resumed, the poison must be eliminated from the system, and the power-producing materials again stored for use.

Stiffness is a form of fatigue due to an accumulation of deposits in the tissues, which are best removed by exercising after a period of rest. With their removal, stiffness disappears, to return with fresh deposits if exercise is again prolonged. The amount of material not taken up by the system lessens with regular exercise, and the tendency to stiffness gradually disappears. The only remedy for stiffness is work, then rest, then work again. Sleep does not always come to the over-tired, and we may therefore conclude that it is better to be rested before attempting to sleep.

A pause, to be recuperative, need not be prolonged; fifteen minutes' rest after exertion should be sufficient; and during a day's work, this fifteen minutes' rest between changes of occupation, not including the quiet necessary for digestion, will keep one fresh. A pause longer than fifteen minutes prepares or readjusts the processes. Do no work, mental or muscular, for at least an hour after a meal; and sleep in a cool—not cold—well-ventilated room.

Low tension power usually accomplishes its object without waste. Work done at high pressure, that might be done at low pressure, indicates waste of effort under strain. The intense concentration of effort when the beginner is struggling with a bicycle is made at high pressure. The excitement of the unexpected probably has something to do with this, as well as the novelty of the situation. If all bicycle work required the same state of tension, however, it could not be long endured; the strain would be too great.

There is a certain amount you can do, or think you can do; this is one measure of your capacity. The work you do is done by stored energy. How may that energy be applied to give the best results? The intricate workings of the mind we may not attempt to analyze: what we do, we do because we wish to, or because we ought, or because we must. Concentrated effort, persistent effort, continuous effort, all consume force. When you dread anything you have undertaken as too difficult of accomplishment, just so much more force is required to overcome that idea. If, mounted on your bicycle, you wheel along in a state of apprehension, you induce a high nervous tension that requires a great reserve of power to resist and supply. Fear, or a sense of insecurity, or a lack of confidence, produces the same result. A bicycle is run by the direct application of power; and power diverted is power wasted.

In wheeling, after the invigorating freshness of the exercise has reached a certain point, the benefit derived lessens with the amount of power drawn from the reserve. Bicycle exercise, moreover, to be really beneficial, should be alternated with other exercise. The bicycle freshens and brings into good condition muscles already developed, but it is an exercise that must be taken with judgment. It is not a panacea for all human ills; it can be generally beneficial, or, immoderately indulged, may become most harmful.

Wheeling for long distances should not be undertaken without proper training. For the sedentary, and for all others tempted by the fascinations of the sport to over-exertion, caution is most necessary. Reaction from over-exertion will bring about a physical condition as detrimental as that caused by lack of exercise—general lassitude and unfitness for work, if nothing more serious.

Persons who are naturally timid cannot accomplish in the same time as much as the more courageous, for their powers are actively at work overcoming their dread of collision and fear of falling; and the distance covered, for power expended, must consequently be less than when no other exertion is required than is needed for propelling the bicycle.

Learn to work without strain or effort; practise where fear is not likely to be aroused, for fear induces a state of tension, and bicycling cannot be enjoyed or prolonged if this drain of the power-supply is allowed. Confidence will come with the knowledge that you are no longer at the mercy of the machine, that it is in your power.

No one make of bicycle is acknowledged the best, and no one is absolutely perfect. The selection of a bicycle, therefore, is a matter of knowledge and nice discrimination, and its use opens a wide field of opportunity before you—touring and cruising, and expeditions of all kinds; travel and sight-seeing; means for study and investigation.

The possible cost of cycling may be quite appalling to consider; but in cycling, as in other things, you may choose between the demands of necessity and the suggestions of luxury. One—almost the chief—fascination of the sport is its simplicity as a mode of travel; the possibility of doing away with all impedimenta. The bicyclist soon learns to dispense with every accessory not positively necessary and to know every possible use of indispensable articles.

The bicycle bestows and restores health; it has its limit, though it does so much that more seems always possible. Take the bicycle as it is, use it intelligently, enjoy it, and become an enthusiast.

About Maria E. Ward

Maria E. Ward (1863–1941), known by her nickname Violet, was an avid bicyclist, the cofounder of the Staten Island Bicycling Club, and the author of *Bicycling for Ladies*. Ward was born in Manhattan, New York, the daughter of General William Greene Ward and Emily Graham Ward, and later lived in Staten Island with her parents and sister. She cofounded the Staten Island Bicycle Club with her friend, the acclaimed photographer Alice Austen, in 1895, and Austen's photographs were used as references for the illustrations in *Bicycling for Ladies*, originally published by Brentano's in 1896 under the name *The Common Sense of Bicycling, Bicycling for Ladies: With Hints as to* *the Art of Wheeling–Advice to Beginners–Dress–Care of the Bicycle–Mechanics–Training–Exercise, etc. etc.*

Ward has been widely celebrated for her contribution to the bicycling world in a wealth of media, including the *New York Times* article "Bicycle Diaries: Two Centuries of New York City History," the *Bust* magazine article "First The Bicycle, Next The Vote: The Story Of Bicycles And Feminism," the book *Mothers and Daughters of Invention*, and *Momentum Mag*, which called her one of the three women "who changed the course of history on bicycles." Ward lived in New York, and died in 1941 at the age of seventy-eight.